SLEEP HACKS

Keith Barry is a world-famous brain hacker and hypnotist and has worked with many world-class athletes, business people, influencers and actors as a mind coach, assisting them to unleash their subconscious potential. His book for adults, *Brain Hacks,* and his book for kids, *Mind Magic,* were both bestsellers.

SLEEP HACKS

KEITH BARRY

DISCOVER THE LIFE-CHANGING TRANQUILLITY OF DEEP SLEEP

Gill Books

Gill Books
Hume Avenue
Park West
Dublin 12
www.gillbooks.ie

Gill Books is an imprint of M.H. Gill and Co.

© Keith Barry 2024

9781804580394

Designed by Bartek Janczak
Print origination by Typo•glyphix
Edited by Claire O'Mahony
Copyedited by Jane Rogers
Printed and bound in Great Britain by Clays Ltd, Elcograf S.p.A.
This book is typeset in Minion Pro.

The content of this book is for information purposes only.
Readers should review the information carefully with their professional healthcare provider. The information is not intended to replace medical advice offered by doctors.

The paper used in this book comes from the wood pulp of sustainably managed forests.

All rights reserved.
No part of this publication may be copied, reproduced or transmitted in any form or by any means, without written permission of the publishers.

A CIP catalogue record for this book is available from the British Library.

5 4 3 2 1

For Mairead, Braden and Breanna.
Your support helped fuel this journey
into the realm of dreams.

CONTENTS

Foreword by Rory Best   ix
Introduction   xi

*

1 Discovering Your Reason 'Why' You Need Better Sleep   1

PART 1: PHYSICAL   29

2 Resetting Your Rhythm   31
3 Feed Your Brain: Eat Well to Sleep Well   53
4 The Glowing Orb of Relaxation   73

PART 2: PSYCHOLOGICAL   95

5 Look into My Eyes   97
6 The Magic of the Black Balloon   115
7 Mind Wipe   135

PART 3: HYPNOMAGICAL   153

8 The Dreambound Descent   155
9 The Sleepscape Garden   177
10 Out-of-Body Sleep   195

11 Closing Questions   215
12 Just for Children!   221

*

Acknowledgements   237
Notes   239

FOREWORD

By Rory Best, former rugby union player and captain of the Ireland national team from 2016 to 2019.

When I first met Keith Barry, little did I know that he would become the key to unlocking a solution to a long-standing challenge I faced – my sleep issue. As an athlete and leader, quality rest and recovery were paramount, but for years I struggled to find the tranquillity of deep sleep. Then came Keith and his remarkable expertise in hypnosis.

In a single session, Keith guided me through a transformative experience, unravelling the busy thoughts that had been hindering my rest for so long. His unique approach to hypnosis not only calmed my racing mind but also taught me valuable techniques to maintain a sense of inner calm even during highly pressurised moments on the pitch.

It wasn't just the immediate effects that amazed me, but the lasting impact it had on my overall wellbeing. Sleep is not just about closing your eyes and waking up the next morning; it's about rejuvenation and mental clarity, and it's the foundation for peak performance. Keith's dedication to helping others and his passion for exploring the untapped power of the mind are evident in every word he speaks and every strategy he imparts.

This book is a testament to Keith's commitment to sharing his knowledge and empowering people to reclaim their sleep and, in turn, their lives. As you delve into the pages ahead, I hope you find the same inspiration and life-changing insights that I did.

INTRODUCTION

Welcome to your new world of better and improved sleep.

As I write this introduction, many different ideas and concepts spring to mind that I could start with. But really the question that needs to be answered first and foremost for you, the reader, is: Why trust me, Keith Barry, to be your sleep guide?

Before getting into the intricacies of sleep hacking, you are most likely wondering why I am qualified to guide you on this journey to improved sleep. As a brain hacker, scientist and hypnotist, I have spent years exploring the complexities of the human mind. Half of my work involves hacking brains purely for entertainment and the other half is concerned with deciphering the subconscious in order to help people create meaningful, sustainable change in connection with their thoughts, behaviours, emotions and, most important for you, their sleep patterns.

I have assisted countless individuals seeking improvement in their lives, and with every single one of them I have noticed a common theme – the profound impact of the intricate relationship between the physical body, conscious mind and subconscious mind on sleep quality. Through my unique approach, blending hypnosis, neuroscience and brain hacking techniques, I have successfully helped many people break free from the shackles of insomnia and sleep disturbance. It's not just some theoretical thing for me; I've actually walked the walk with hundreds, if not thousands, of people. My aim is to help everyone, including me, achieve a better quality of life through improved sleep.

This is no ordinary sleep book. I'll be sharing many stories from my life and I'll also share techniques I have developed that may seem to go beyond your current understanding of reality. My purpose is to give you an insight into these techniques and how they originated.

I want this book to be an authentic reflection of my work, so I have designed, researched or extensively tested everything in these pages. While the majority of the techniques in this book align with current neuroscience, some of them are based on my expertise in the world of the unconscious mind, which is massively complex.

I am 100 per cent confident that the system in this book works. I aspire to someday put my work under even more scientific scrutiny, through trials that will help bridge the gap between my current knowledge and that of the scientific community.

The current sleep challenges that people face seem worse than ever. Since Covid-19, my website has been inundated with people reporting their struggles in achieving a good night's sleep. The struggle is real, but you must accept that the end of your personal struggle starts today. Right here. Right now. In this moment.

If you are still contemplating whether this book is for you, please answer these three key questions:

1. Do I acknowledge that sleep is one of the most important aspects of my life and am I prepared to dedicate the attention necessary to improve the quality of my sleep?
2. Am I willing to trust Keith and the insights he presents in this book?
3. Am I committed to not just reading but studying this book and actively trying and applying the strategies until I see a positive shift in my sleep patterns?

If the answer to these three questions is Yes, please read on. If the answer is No, put the book down and don't waste any more of your time.

HOW TO USE THIS BOOK

THE MYSTERY OF SLEEP

Sleep is a universal experience, yet it remains a mainly mysterious phenomenon. It's only in recent years that scientists have begun to understand sleep and its importance for our mental and physical health. Why is it that one person can effortlessly drift into a deep slumber, while another battles in the grip of insomnia? What sets apart those who wake up refreshed from those who stumble through their day burdened by fatigue? Why does one person wake in the middle of the night multiple times while another sleeps soundly all night long? Why do some people function on low amounts of sleep while others need a full eight hours' sleep in order to get through their day?

These questions have fuelled my exploration into the world of sleep, which has led me to a revelation: the answers lie in three key areas which we will explore together and use to formulate a system to aid your sleep:

1. **Physical:** You will explore a variety of methods that you can use to prepare your physical body for a good night's sleep. By prioritising your physical wellbeing, you are setting the stage for priming yourself for success.
2. **Psychological:** You will learn how to declutter your conscious mind and how to release worries and concerns in preparation for deep relaxation. By releasing those worries and cultivating a calm mental space you will pave the way towards a rejuvenating night's sleep.
3. **Hypnomagical:** You will discover how to hack your subconscious mind to help you drift off into a deep sleep on a nightly basis. You will use self-hypnosis to guide your subconscious mind towards deep sleep.

The subconscious mind is really the world's first supercomputer and you have the ability to input, extract and even delete information, once you know how. The subconscious holds the key to understanding and transforming our sleep patterns. I've spent my entire adult life hacking both my own subconscious mind and the subconscious minds of other people, with truly transformative results. I truly believe that if you commit wholeheartedly to the techniques in this book, which have evolved over the last three decades (that makes my bones shiver – I can't believe I've been doing this that long), your sleep will definitely improve. That's why you can trust me.

In this book you get to design your own sleep system. This is not a one-size-fits-all strategy. Although 99.99 per cent of our DNA is the same, you are unique and you need to find a system that is unique to you. The good news is that the system is super easy to create.

My ask right now is very simple, and one I will remind you of again throughout the book.

There are 21 different Sleep Hacks contained in these pages, divided between the book's three sections – Physical, Psychological and Hypnomagical.

I want you to choose three hacks and use them for 30 days:

> - **One** from the **Physical** section (Sleep Hacks 1–6)
> - **One** from the **Psychological** section (Sleep Hacks 7–15)
> - **One** from the **Hypnomagical** section (Sleep Hacks 16–21)

Use these in combination for a month, and if by the end of the month you are still struggling with your sleep, swap one of the hacks for another in the same category.

There are also 'Try this' information boxes, and these are simply extra suggestions or tips that you can decide to use or not.

Where a Sleep Hack has several steps to it, I've included a quick recap at the end, where you can quickly remind yourself how to do it without having to read the entire chapter.

Can you do more than three Sleep Hacks? Of course! You can do as many as you like, but start by doing the three you chose, one from each section.

Learning through repetition is key. You may see a profound improvement after just one day, but most likely the improvement will come after a number of days or weeks.

As a scientist I've always loved formulae. The following is a straightforward formula I designed that encapsulates the essence of the journey you are about to take. Spend some moments thinking about the elements in the formula and why they are there. Understand that if you follow this formula, your quest for improved sleep will be achieved much easier and also faster.

$$(D + M) \times SH = IS$$

Let's break it down:

> - Desire (**D**): The first step towards transforming your sleep patterns is cultivating a strong desire for change. Take a moment to recognise the importance of quality sleep in your life and acknowledge the impact it has on your overall wellbeing.
> - Motivation (**M**): Coupled with desire, motivation fuels the engine of change. Understand the benefits that improved sleep can bring to your physical, mental and emotional health. Use this motivation as a driving force to embark on the journey of sleep hacking.
> - Sleep Hacks (**SH**): Armed with the desire and motivation for change, it's time to explore an arsenal of sleep hacks. These hacks encompass a range of techniques, from relaxation exercises to self-hypnosis strategies, tailored to address the specific nuances of your subconscious sleep patterns.
> - Improved Sleep (**IS**): The combination of desire, motivation and sleep hacks leads to the ultimate goal – improved sleep. Imagine waking up each morning feeling refreshed, energised and ready to conquer the day. This is the promise of *Sleep Hacks*.

YOUR JOURNEY

In the pages that follow, we will delve deep into the intricacies of sleep hacking, exploring the science behind subconscious programming, unveiling practical techniques and sharing real-life success stories.

By the end of this journey, you not only will understand the mechanics of your sleep patterns but will also possess the tools to rewire your brain for a restful and rejuvenating night's sleep.

1

DISCOVERING YOUR REASON 'WHY' YOU NEED BETTER SLEEP

DISCOVERING YOUR 'SUBCONSCIOUS WHY'

Why is it that you need better sleep? That's the first question I get people to ask themselves before I give them any sleep improvement technique. Your immediate conscious answer is most likely, 'Jaysus, Barry, you're a bit thick – it's obvious! I'm not sleeping great and I'm tired as a result.' It's a basic question, you might think, but it's a necessary one: you must define what it is you're looking to achieve by getting more sleep so that you can change your behaviours and commit to improving your habits. Your habits and behaviours are ingrained in your subconscious, so in order to create meaningful, permanent change you need to peel back the layers of grey matter and mine deep for your subconscious 'why'.

Everybody reading this book will have a different reason for picking it up. Someone might feel anxious and they know that it's linked to their poor sleep. Other people will be aware of the many studies showing that living longer is linked with good sleep. Maybe you're looking to be more productive or less bad-tempered, or you want to look sexier for your Instagram feed. You more than likely know the conscious reason you picked up this book, but what I want you to do is to identify the subconscious reason why you're reading it. It's necessary for you to spend some time digging deep and finding the real reason you want better sleep in order for the system that follows to work for you.

I've already asked you to pick three techniques from each section of the book. Alongside that, I'm asking you to discover your subconscious reason for sleep.

DIGGING DEEP

Here is how to discover your subconscious 'why'. This technique may seem unusual or crazy, but trust me when I say I've helped hundreds of people find their inner 'why' for sleep improvement using this technique:

1. Find a quiet, safe space where you can comfortably relax, either sitting or lying down.
2. Close your eyes and breathe in through your nose and out through your mouth deeply 10 times. Breathe in for 4 seconds, hold for 2 seconds, and exhale for 4 seconds. Now clear your mind and begin to imagine you are floating in outer space. Let go of all the tension in your physical body as you enjoy the

feeling of weightlessness. Add in the details of the spacesuit you are wearing and begin to notice the planets and stars all around you. Ensure you take some time to fully invest your imagination into the process.

3. Notice now a space station in front of you. This is a serene and safe place that represents the higher consciousness of your subconscious mind. With curiosity and intrigue, float towards the space station and open the door. Float inside and notice that this space is filled with images, symbols, words, drawings and emotions. Allow yourself to think freely with no inhibitions and allow your subconscious mind to play within the psychological safety of your own mind. Take your time to allow these thoughts to generate from your subconscious mind.

4. As you float through the space station remember what resonates with you as being most important.

5. Ask yourself many questions as you float through the space, beginning only with the words 'why' or 'what'. For example: What is my deeper purpose here? Why is it that I need more energy? Why is it I need to rest my body and mind with deep sleep? Why did I buy this book? What activities am I struggling with right now that could benefit from better sleep? What is it about *that* image that brings up *this* emotion?

6. As you continue to explore the answers to these questions, notice what other images, symbols, words and pictures come to mind. Since this is a creative subconscious exploration, give yourself the freedom to allow zany, crazy thoughts, pictures, words and images to enter your mind.

7. Trust the process, knowing your subconscious mind is seeking the answers you desire.

8. Now imagine a bridge from the space station to the physical space where you are currently sitting or lying down. Visualise the astronaut version of yourself floating back into the present version of yourself, bringing the newly found subconscious answers back to your conscious mind to explore.
9. When you are ready, open your eyes and reflect on the experience.
10. Write down all the answers you can remember from your exploration in a notebook and reflect on them by continuing to ask more 'what' and 'why' questions.

When doing this, I always advise people to go at least ten layers down into their subconscious 'why' and 'what' questions; in other words you should ask a minimum of ten of those types of question. However, there's no limit as to how far you can mine down into your subconscious mind. It could take you just a single session to do this or it may take multiple sessions, but if you keep mining for an answer that you have never thought about before you will *always* get a revelation. When that revelation happens, everything will change for the better and give you the motivation necessary to improve your sleep habits. What do I mean? I'll give you my story as an example.

WHY I DECIDED I NEEDED BETTER SLEEP

I sought out better sleep because I wanted to be more productive and get more things done. Superficially, it's as simple as that.

During one of my own personal space station explorations (you should do this many times, as you will go deeper and deeper into your subconscious the more you do it) I saw dozens and dozens of images, beings, pictures, sketches, words, sentences and drawings.

Flying wallabies, underground fantastical gardens, floating libraries, bioluminescent flying insects, a party with my friends in Vegas where I was aged 150, and more! I chose to zone in on images that I saw of my children, salmon that were floating around my head, and a movie on a screen in the space station where I saw myself aged 90 with my wife and grandkids swimming at Derrynane beach in Kerry. I zoned in on the swimming and salmon images and asked myself:

Why is it that there was salmon in that space station and why was I 90 years old swimming with my wife? *Because I love fishing for salmon and swimming in the sea but don't ever have enough time to get around to either.*

Why is fishing important? *It's my way to unwind and empty my brain, and it's cheaper than therapy.*

Why is sea swimming important? *I feel at peace in the sea and rejuvenated afterwards.*

What would life look like if I fished or swam more? *I'd be more relaxed and more creative.*

The first few layers down is the easy part, but then you have to push further.

What would you create as a result of being more creative? *I'd create a legacy.*

Why is a legacy important? *To make my kids proud.*

What would a legacy look like? *I've no idea.*

After much reflection and 42 layers in, this is what my revelation is:

I'd clean up the rivers and seas to help with the decline in wild Atlantic salmon stocks (according to Inland Fisheries Ireland, they're down about 70 per cent from just thirty years ago) and to create a healthy sea swimming environment for my kids and grandkids when I am 90.

You keep pushing and pushing and pushing, digging and mining, and what eventually happens is that a revelation will come from your subconscious.

I worked all the way down into the legacy I'd like to leave behind when I die as a result of my subconscious mind revealing to me what I am passionate about, and those two things are fishing and the sea. I'd like to leave a healthy river and sea system behind. At the time of writing this, there are 32 raw sewage pipes pumping untreated sewage into the seas all around Ireland, something that a lot of people aren't aware of. Everybody will tell you that it's an impossible problem to solve because it's a multi-billion euro problem. Last year I turned 47, and as a result of my subconscious revelation my aim is to be financially free by the time I'm 55. The reason I want to be financially free is because that gives me ten years to the conventional retirement age of 65 or so (even though I'll never retire) to get all 32 raw sewage pipes either fixed or shut down. I'm giving myself ten years from 55 to 65 to focus and zone in on shutting down all 32 raw sewage pipes all around Ireland. It is impractical for me right now to do this because I've got so much going on and I don't have the resources of time and effort and energy. It's a full-time commitment. That's why I need to be financially free. And now I know. I know I simply *must* gain enough sleep nightly to be mega-productive every day. It becomes effortless because I am motivated by my new-found subconscious purpose.

This is the reason and the driving force behind why I seek and find great sleep. I have a long-term plan that I am passionate about and excited at a deep neurological level about achieving.

Of course, 99.99 per cent of the people I've mentioned this to have told me that cleaning up or shutting down all 32 raw sewage pipes is an impossible problem to solve. Those opinions actually help me. They give me fuel to know that, in the words of Audrey Hepburn, impossible simply means 'I'm Possible', and I'm 100 per cent certain that this is my defined internal purpose. Nothing and no one will stop me.

You too need to find your own subconscious reason why you need more sleep, because once you identify that, you will never stop until you achieve great sleep on a regular basis. It doesn't need to be as grandiose as my own vision, but you do need to find and define it. Once you find your revelation, deep in your subconscious, your path becomes clearer and your journey to sleep becomes easier.

I did this with a client recently, and when his revelation happened, he bawled his eyes out with joy for five minutes straight. Tom is a 42-year-old business owner from Galway, with a wife and one young child. He has not slept more than five to six hours for approximately 15 years. His session went something like this:

Tom, tell me what you saw while floating around your space station.

I saw a rollercoaster made from spaghetti, family Polaroid photos from the future floating in space, homeless people eating in a restaurant in the Eiffel Tower, a Lego robot, the world being dominated by cyborgs ... and many more images, concepts and ideas. It was interesting but none of it makes any sense.

What concepts were the strongest in your mind and gave you the most emotion?

The homeless image and the image of cyborgs.

Why do you think you saw homeless people?

Because when I was 22 years old I was homeless for six months.

Why did that happen?

I was abusing alcohol at the time and had no respect for myself or the ones I loved.

What did you learn from that experience?

To always have empathy for other people and never judge them.

Why do you think an image of cyborgs came up?

Because I understand AI (Tom owns a software firm) *and the fact is that I believe cyborgs will become a reality for us all very soon.*

What feeling did that give you?

I felt scared and uncertain.

I kept digging and mining with Tom and eventually a revelation happened – keep reading to find out what that revelation was!

You may discover more than one subconscious 'why' when looking for the real reason why you need better and more sleep. I realised this during the period when I didn't sleep well for almost a year. I found that lack of sleep made me cranky, with less tolerance for other people. I could be quite sharp with them, which is not in my true personality, and I didn't like this behaviour; that isn't the type of person I wanted to be. I wanted to move away from this behaviour as fast as possible. The behaviour bothered me because I wasn't living true to my values.

Once again, I returned to the space station and back to the 'why'. Why is it important that I live true to my values? Because I understand that my life is defined by my values. Those values change over time for me, but right now, they include curiosity, integrity, authenticity, adventure, compassion and empathy. What is it about my life that would look different if I lived by my defined values? I'd have more success, professionally and personally. I'd be more content. I would have better connections with my loved ones. I'd have a deeper sense of fulfilment. I'd realise I am enough as I am.

And guess what? When you are living a life aligned with your highest values your sleep will automatically improve, as you will be living an authentic and fulfilled existence.

How do you find your highest values and live a life defined by them? Simply by putting in some thought into what they are! When was the last time you nailed down your values and committed to living your life aligned to those values?

DEFINING YOUR VALUES FOR LIFE

Read the following list and write down or circle the five values that resonate with you the most. If there is a value that comes to mind that isn't on the list, feel free to add it.

1. Integrity
2. Honesty
3. Respect
4. Responsibility
5. Accountability
6. Compassion
7. Empathy
8. Fairness
9. Trustworthiness
10. Authenticity
11. Loyalty
12. Gratitude
13. Generosity
14. Humility

15. Patience
16. Perseverance
17. Courage
18. Open-mindedness
19. Tolerance
20. Flexibility
21. Collaboration
22. Teamwork
23. Excellence
24. Innovation
25. Creativity
26. Passion
27. Determination
28. Self-discipline
29. Self-awareness
30. Self-improvement
31. Growth
32. Learning
33. Curiosity
34. Balance
35. Harmony
36. Diversity
37. Inclusivity
38. Sustainability
39. Environmental stewardship
40. Community involvement
41. Social justice
42. Equality
43. Empowerment

44. Independence
45. Freedom
46. Commitment
47. Open communication
48. Adaptability
49. Resilience
50. Quality

Now commit to living your life fully aligned to those values. Never compromise. If you do this, you'll find contentment and as a result not only will your sleep improve but your whole life will improve. Live your life by design, not by accident.

Everyone's subconscious 'why' and core values are going to be different. It's important that you keep pushing and pushing, and that you don't settle for the easy answer when mining for your subconscious 'why'. You need to find that revelation, and it's not a process to be rushed, so make sure you set aside the time to do it and keep mining, mining, mining. And remember, do it at least five times to truly allow your conscious mind to settle and your subconscious mind to provide you with the answers you desire.

I bet you're still wondering what Tom's subconscious 'why' turned out to be.

It's as follows:

I want to create a portable technology device designed specifically for homeless people to help them access essential services and resources.

He cried and cried when he told me. I asked him why he was so emotional. He responded by saying he had just been clocking in and out for years with no real motivation or sense of purpose. He was just plodding along and getting through life, as so many people tend to do. He was certain that this revelation was his new subconscious 'why'. He is now fully committed to doing everything necessary to achieving that new-found purpose, including improving his quality of sleep.

Once you've completed the above process, you're almost ready to design your own sleep system from the techniques in this book.

CULTIVATING DISCIPLINE (IT'S NOT AS BAD AS IT SOUNDS)

Before you begin any of the techniques, we need to tackle the most boring word in the world but perhaps the most important – discipline. When it comes to sleep the most essential ask I'll have of you is to maintain your discipline when you begin to use the techniques in this book. Discipline plays a crucial role in the intricate machinery of attaining consistent and peaceful sleep. It's the unsung hero that, when applied consistently, can lead to a profound transformation in your sleep patterns.

When you commit to practising three Sleep Hack techniques from this book you must be disciplined enough to use them daily for a minimum of 30 days in order to assess whether or not they work for you.

Of course, you can always go with the 'Sleep when you're dead' mindset, which will actually work earlier than expected for you if that's the way you choose to mentally programme yourself. There's over fifty years of scientific evidence of the link between sleep duration and mortality; as early as 1964, data indicated that those who achieved 7 hours of sleep had the lowest risk for all mortality, while those who deviated from 7–8 hours – both those who slept the shortest and the longest – have significantly higher mortality risk. But since you're reading this book I'll assume you've already eliminated the 'sleep when you're dead' thought process.

The enemy of discipline is our ego – we must put our ego aside and understand we are all on a similar yet different path. We are similar in that we all share the inevitable, we're all on a journey to the grave, and most of us decide to push that thought to the back of our mind. Yet we are different enough that some of us focus on our physical health for longevity and some also focus on our mental health. Others don't bat an eyelid over either, and for many of those people there is no changing them. But you are here to change for the better. You must understand and trust me when I say the number one focus in your life should be your sleep. It's easy to not think about death. It's easier to think we are invincible. It's easier to choose short-term satisfaction over long-term gains because we like to think we will live for ever. I'm not scaremongering by any means, but just make the decision now that if you put in the discipline necessary to cure or aid your sleep, you are adding days, months or even potentially years to your life. Don't leave it to chance. Decide right now to take my 30-day challenge – and that 30-day challenge may indeed change your life for ever.

I CHALLENGE YOU TO A 30-DAY DISCIPLINE CHALLENGE!

In a world characterised by instant gratification, the concept of discipline may seem tedious, or even archaic. Yet, it remains an indispensable tool in the quest for better sleep. The commitment to discipline is especially crucial when adopting the techniques outlined in this book.

I asked you to take the following action in the introduction, but in case you missed it or skipped the introduction, here it is again:

Commit fully to using three of the 21 Sleep Hack techniques, one from each section – Physical, Psychological and Hypnomagical – for the next 30 days.

What I love about this book is that you get to create a system that works for you. The system is very simple. Combine and use one technique from each section and that becomes your system for the month.

While this book doesn't offer a miracle cure, it does contain many solutions that will work for most people. There is no excuse here. Discipline is the key to unlocking your journey to attaining regular, peaceful sleep.

Let's set the record straight – there is no magic sprinkle and no wave of a magic wand which will get you to sleep. No magic pill. The real magic lies inside you and rests in the discipline necessary to reset your mind and body to follow the natural rhythm of sleep. Commitment is the key in order to reset yourself to do what your body and mind naturally know how to do.

Choose three techniques, one from each section in the book:

> One from **Physical** (Sleep Hacks 1–6)
> One from **Psychological** (Sleep Hacks 7–15)
> One from **Hypnomagical** (Sleep Hacks 16–21).

When you choose a combination of techniques from this book, give them at least 30 days of constant practice. This timeline is not random; it aligns with the time it takes for the mind and body to adapt to new routines and habits. If after a month you are in the unlikely situation that you have seen no improvement, don't become disheartened. Instead, be disciplined enough to try another technique or combination of techniques for another 30 days.

Every single morning, I joyfully shout to my kids 'NGU!', which means Never Give Up. Decide right here right now that this is the beginning of the end of your journey with your sleep struggles. There are enough techniques in this book for every single person to find a solution. But you must decide right now to NGU – if you need to try every single solution in this book, so be it. If it takes three months, so be it. If it takes longer, that's okay too. NGU and discipline are your friends.

So ask yourself right now:

> How disciplined am I?
> Do I try something for a day and if it doesn't work will I stop?
> Do I try something for a week but if it doesn't work I'll stop?

A lot of the time, when people fail it's because of their lack of discipline. Of course, there can be other reasons too, but a lack of discipline will always cause you to fail.

Imagine for a moment your mind is like a vault in a bank. However, instead of storing cash or gold, I want you to lock your desire to sleep deep into your mind vault. No one and nothing can access your vault. Not even you, because you've forgotten the combination. Any time a thought or desire comes to mind that conflicts with your desire to sleep, consider that an attack on your vault. However, accept that it is impenetrable and the moment the attack happens you will be able to deflect that thought immediately, whether it's your own thought or someone else's.

THE INSTANT GRATIFICATION DILEMMA

Everything in the modern era has become instant. In a world accustomed to instant solutions – coffee at the push of a button, groceries being delivered to our front door, cars that drive themselves, even packages dropped by drone into our back garden – our brains have become lazy with all these shortcuts and immediate rewards: *Got a headache? Take a pill. Need to get to the third floor of a building? Use an elevator. Want a fast meal? Use a microwave. Finding it hard to sleep? Take some sleeping tablets.* There is a problem with all of this. Our brains have become dumbed down and we expect a quick fix for everything.

Try this the next time you think about doing something that you know will affect your sleep cycle. Imagine it's a Thursday night and you've had a very productive week. You start thinking: *I deserve a glass of wine. Sure it's good for me and it's nearly the weekend anyway.* Many people will fight with that thought for a moment but then automatically open the bottle of wine anyhow. If you don't drink, the thought could be another one that conflicts with sleep, like binge watching a TV show. The next time you get a thought like this that you know will affect your sleep, begin practising my sleepguard strategy:

TRY THIS: THE SLEEPGUARD STRATEGY

When a thought enters your head that conflicts with your desire for improving your sleep, you must shut down that thought immediately. Here's a great hack for doing just that. The moment the thought comes to mind simply use both thumbs to touch your other four fingers, one at a time, starting with your index finger. As you touch the index finger say silently to yourself 'sleep'. Now, as you touch your middle finger, say silently 'matters', then 'more' with your third finger, and finally 'defend' when you touch your little finger. Do this three times in total so you have said the sentence 'Sleep matters more, defend.' Notice how that intrusive thought gets pushed away into the distance as you guard your inner sleep vault. Give that thought no more significance as it fades away.

REPROGRAMMING THE LAZY BRAIN

To embark on the journey towards deep and rejuvenating sleep we need to reprogram our minds to maintain our discipline throughout that journey.

So let's start with a problem we all have. Thinking about tomorrow. Our conscious and subconscious minds are like washing machines of ideas and concepts preparing for tomorrow, but when the world moves so fast and we have so many activities and information to deal with it all seems overwhelming.

THE 'MONKEY MIND' AND PLANNING FOR TOMORROW

As I write this chapter, I'm on a plane to London, juggling a messy life between live and virtual performances, family responsibilities and other commitments. I'm flying over to give a motivational speech. My sleep wasn't optimal last night and I know I won't be at my best today. Let's dissect for a moment why that might be. I think it's important when writing a book like this that I pull back the curtains a few times in order for you to realise that although my sleep is really good now, I still have nights when it just doesn't seem to work out. We must be kind to ourselves on this quest and understand that failure is okay as long as we learn quickly from those failures.

I went to bed late after a performance last night. I did some things you'll learn from the book to optimise my sleep: I ate two kiwis; I read a book. I used the Magic of the Black Balloon technique, which you'll read about in a subsequent chapter. It seemed I did everything right. *But* the rest of the household was still awake. I could hear the kids and my wife and no matter what I say to them, they are incapable of being quiet. I made the rookie mistake of not putting in earplugs or using noise-cancelling headphones. Then I randomly woke up in the middle of the night with freezing cold feet! That's a first for me and I wondered should I wear socks to bed. When I investigated this, I found studies that indicate that wearing socks to bed can indeed help with your sleep.[1] This is because wearing socks increases blood circulation to your feet, and as a result your blood vessels widen. Consequently, your core body temperature is lowered, and this process leads to a more rapid onset of sleep. If it happens again, I'm definitely going to start wearing socks in bed.

Now, on to tomorrow. I will be back home in Ireland to deliver a virtual motivational speech from my home studio. This is completely different from the live event in London today and requires adequate planning. I also have to bring my son to a rugby match and I have a meeting in the evening. Then I'll visit my parents for dinner. And lots more in between.

Here's the rub – if I leave everything to chance, with zero planning, my monkey mind will switch on when I go to the leaba and my mind will whir, knowingly or unknowingly, all night long. The term 'monkey mind' originates in Buddhism and it means a mind that is unsettled, confused and flitting from thought to thought.

Maybe that's why I woke up and it wasn't the cold feet. I'm not sure. What I do know is that although I did some things correctly, I didn't fully maintain my discipline; I didn't make plans for today and write them down. That's why right now I'm going to plan for tomorrow.

PLANNING IS THE ANTIDOTE

So in just a moment I'll be logging off my computer and going to the Notes app on my phone in order to begin planning for the next 12 hours.

Here is what I know I'll be writing down:

- Set alarm for 7.30 a.m.
- Breathwork immediately in bed for 15 minutes followed by 15 minutes' creative visualisation
- 8 a.m. – Prepare ice bath
- 8.10–8.30 a.m. – Grounding (the therapeutic technique where you physically reconnect with the earth), either in the back garden or using an electromagnetic PEMF mat – more on this later
- 8.30 a.m. – Ice bath for four minutes
- 8.45 a.m. – Shower and get dressed, ready to attack the day
- 9–10.30 a.m. – Prepare for the virtual show
- 10.30–11 a.m. – Coffee break
- 11 a.m. – 12.30 p.m. – Virtual show
- 12.30–2 p.m. – Gym
- 2–3 p.m. – Lunch
- 3–4 p.m. – Dreaded Zoom meetings
- 4 p.m. – Collect my daughter from school

- 5–6 p.m. – Family time including chess with my daughter and Xbox with my son (I love gaming with my son!)
- 6–7.30 p.m. – Snack; then bring my son to rugby
- 8 p.m. – Dinner with my wife and folks
- 9–10.30 p.m. – Begin the process of winding down for sleep
- 11 p.m. – Bed

The silver lining is I have a 'focus' system for planning. When you map out your day, your mind will quieten. This is because it wants order. As humans we are all pattern-seekers and pattern-followers, and the order created by planning helps to quieten the monkey mind. Granted, some people thrive in chaos, but a lot of us, myself included, love order. That's why writing down my list of things to do and having a plan offloads some of the stress from my brain and allows me to focus on sleep. One study found that people who wrote to-do lists fell asleep nine minutes sooner than people who wrote about their previous day's accomplishments, and the more specific the lists were, the sooner they fell asleep.[2] It mightn't sound like much of a win, but the researchers noted that nine minutes is approximately the same as it takes sleep medications to work.

FOCUS: THE ART OF UNVEILING DISCIPLINE

I have a fondness for order, and I love using acronyms to help people remember strategies. I'd like to introduce you to my FOCUS acronym, which is designed to assist you in always focusing the spotlight on your discipline.

THE POWER OF DISCIPLINE

In the wonderful world of magic, discipline acts as the invisible hand that transforms a mere trick into an awe-inspiring spectacle. As someone who has dedicated a lifetime to perfecting the art of illusion, I've come to realise that discipline is not merely a tool – it's the underlying secret behind every seamless performance.

During my *Magic Madhouse* tour, I performed an underwater illusion every single night on stage for 30 nights. It involved me getting shackled and chained with stainless steel handcuffs and restraints and then I was trapped in a tank of water from which I had to escape. I succeeded in escaping every single night, not because I'm the best escapologist in the world, or the best illusionist. I succeeded because I had the discipline necessary to learn how to hold my breath underwater for up to four minutes. I succeeded because I had the discipline necessary to spend countless hours in the months running up to the tour learning how to pick locks with my eyes closed. I also succeeded by having the discipline necessary to get adequate sleep and rest every night to have the energy to perform at my peak on stage for each and every audience.

By the way, at that time I had a very interesting way to prepare for sleep. Think about it logically – I would be on stage every night for two-and-a-half hours. Every night I would give it my all, and most nights I would get a standing ovation. I could easily have let that go to my head and celebrated nightly by boozing and dancing the night away. Instead I would drive home and prepare for sleep. To help wind down, I would immediately get into my pjs, have a cup of herbal tea and watch mind-numbing TV, always the same programme – *Judge Judy*! Then I would head to bed, read a book and practise gratitude for the standing ovation. Not very 'rock and roll', but it served me well, and that's because I was following my FOCUS technique, which I developed all the way back in 2003.

> F: Formulate a clear vision
> O: Organise resources
> C: Consistency
> U: Understand the power of adaptability
> S: Stimulate your passion

INITIATING DISCIPLINE: UNVEILING THE ILLUSION

Discipline, much like a magic trick, begins with a moment of inspiration – a decision to embark on a journey of mastery. In the world of magic, this beginning often mirrors the spark that ignites the disciplined pursuit of a difficult manoeuvre – for example the one-handed top palm – a move that requires not only technical precision but also unwavering focus. The one-handed top palm is a sleight of hand technique used in card magic, where the magician conceals a card from the audience's view by palming it with one hand. The magician skilfully hides the card in the palm of their hand while maintaining a natural and relaxed appearance, creating the illusion that the hand is empty when it is actually concealing a card. When it comes to discipline, I reckon there are very few artists who have the discipline or dedication of the magician.

F: FORMULATING A CLEAR VISION

The initiation of discipline demands a clear vision. Going back to my love of sleight of hand, this clarity manifested in the desire to master the difficult one-handed top palm. The journey to perfecting this near-impossible manoeuvre began with understanding what I wanted to achieve – seamless mastery over a complex sleight that would captivate audiences. It also had to be perfected to an extent that the audience would not even know the sleight had occurred.

My vision for the trick that would be achieved using the sleight was also clear – I wanted Irish radio DJ Dave Fanning to sign a playing card and mix it among 3,000 other playing cards, which were then loaded by him into air cannons. I would then be hoisted 150 feet in the air on a crane and would bungee jump off the crane with a sword in my hand and spear his signed card with the tip of the sword. I needed to perfect the one-handed top palm to achieve this. After countless hours dropping cards and going through massive bouts of frustration I perfected the sleight. It wasn't easy. I wanted to give up at times but my desire to achieve the outcome outweighed those moments of frustration. In 2003 Dave appeared on *Close Encounters with Keith Barry* on RTÉ One and I pulled off the trick seamlessly. It is one of my favourite pieces of magic I've ever performed.

Know that your journey may be easy. It may be difficult. But once you have your vision and commit fully to it nothing will stop you. Decide right now what your vision is regarding this book. If you've already done the 'finding your reason why' exercise, you will already know what your long-term goal is. And this can be anything from being less cranky to living a longer life. Once you know what your target is, a great idea is to write it down in the form of a contract with yourself, and then commit to finding joy in the process.

Here's an example of a self-contract:

> I, (your name) _____
> will complete my goal of improving my sleep by following the techniques in this book and commit to designing and following my own system for at least 30 days. I will choose one technique from each section, and if one of these isn't working well for me, I will try another technique from the same section. By doing this, I will be able to move forward in my life, my health and my mental wellbeing, and I will be able to work towards my goals.
>
> I hereby commit to actively focusing on my sleep and achieving better sleep.
>
> Signed: _____

Whether it's executing a magical sleight or adhering to a disciplined routine, infusing joy into the journey is key. Happiness sustains discipline. Just as finding joy in fitness involves enjoying the process of healthy eating and regular exercise, so too you can find joy in your quest for sleep. Enjoy trying out the new techniques in this book – and commit to doing them wholeheartedly until you find a solution that works for you.

O: ORGANISING RESOURCES

Just as a magician organises props and techniques, you must organise the resources necessary for your disciplined journey. Identify the skills or knowledge required. The one-handed top palm, for instance, required a fresh deck of cards as the prop and demanded a deep understanding of card manipulation, hand positioning and audience psychology. For example, if you find a new food in this book that you think you might want to try in order to help your sleep, don't wait. Order it immediately so you are prepared ASAP. If you decide to read before you go to sleep, get that book right now and place it next to your bed. Ensure your room is prepared every night to be sleep-friendly. Make sure you have comfortable sleep attire to slip into before you hit the hay. Prepare, prepare, prepare, and then execute.

C: CONSISTENCY IS PARAMOUNT

Whether executing a complex magic move or adhering to a new sleep routine, discipline thrives on consistency. Small, daily efforts accumulate into significant achievements. Consistency in refining the one-handed top palm ensured a seamless performance each time it was utilised. And that reminds me of one key strategy I ask you now to do every single day:

Make your bed the moment you get out of it.

(Unless of course your partner is still sleeping in the bed because, let's face it, making the bed over their head while they are still sleeping might not go down too well!)

Much has been written about the habit of making your bed first thing in the morning because it will trigger other positive habits. In the motivational book *Make Your Bed* by William H. McCraven, based on life lessons from his Navy SEAL training, he argues that making your bed as soon as you get up is an easy task to achieve, and one that will make you feel more productive, enabling you to jump on to the next task. It starts you off on the right foot.

But I'm asking you to do it for another reason. By making your bed in the morning you are already subliminally telling your subconscious mind that you are preparing for a good night's rest later that evening/night. You are beginning the priming process in your mind to gear up towards a peaceful sleep. You need to respect your sleep space. So treat it accordingly. Most people would not go out to dinner with friends in clothes that were unkempt or untidy – they just wouldn't feel good. Treat your bed with the same respect you treat yourself with and watch the difference that small change can make. It will also encourage you to keep the rest of your bedroom neat and tidy. This is a definite plus if you spend precious minutes in the morning tearing everything asunder to try and find a clean shirt. I'll be looking at the whole area of creating and maintaining a beautiful sleep environment in the next chapter, but the first step in this process is to start making that bed and being consistent with the practice.

U: UNDERSTAND THE POWER OF ADAPTABILITY

Life is dynamic, and so is discipline. Recognise that there will be phases of intensity and moments of lapse in your discipline journey. Adaptability is essential. In magic, adapting to unexpected situations is crucial.

I'm reminded of the time I was tutoring Woody Harrelson to act as the mentalist and hypnotist Merritt in the movie *Now You See Me*. I had taught him a really amazing mind-reading trick to perform on *The David Letterman Show*. Woody had practised the trick and I had agreed with the producers that he would perform the trick using a book I had provided. However, when we arrived the producers said that Letterman insisted that Woody use his (Letterman's) books.

This was absolutely crazy – Letterman was basically challenging Woody to really read his mind. I told the producers that was no problem – Woody would do it with Letterman's books. Woody was shocked – he had no idea how to do what I was saying he could do and he was due on air in 30 minutes. I taught Woody how to do the effect with borrowed books and he went on to destroy Letterman's mind live on air. At the time of writing this you can still find that clip on YouTube.

All the tools and techniques in this book are malleable and adaptable. Use your imagination to tweak them to suit your personal physiology and psychology. Don't want to eat two kiwis? Eat one! Don't want to spend money on an earthing mat? Walk into the back garden barefoot. Don't want to read before bed? No problem. Write instead. Don't want to read *or* write? No problem. Close your eyes and creatively visualise. Struggle with visualisation? No problem. Imagine you can visualise! You have a profound mind – use it to adapt and find what works for you.

S: STIMULATE YOUR PASSION

Much as my love for magic helped me sustain gruelling practice sessions, passion fuels discipline and restful sleep. Just as a magician meticulously hones their skills and dedicates countless hours to perfecting their art, your commitment to prioritising sleep and establishing healthy bedtime routines will be the key to unlocking the magic of rejuvenation and overall wellbeing in your life. Your passion for quality sleep will act as the driving force that transforms each night into a restorative experience, ensuring you wake up each morning refreshed, revitalised and ready to embrace the day with renewed energy and enthusiasm.

Finding that passion is easier than you might think. Once you have discovered your subconscious 'why', by simply immersing yourself wholeheartedly in this book and opening your mind to the vast array of topics discussed, you will uncover a genuine passion for promoting and improving your sleep health.

Once you've digested this chapter, you're ready to embark on the first chapter in the Physical section of the book, where you will learn how to prime your body for a great night's sleep.

PART 1: PHYSICAL

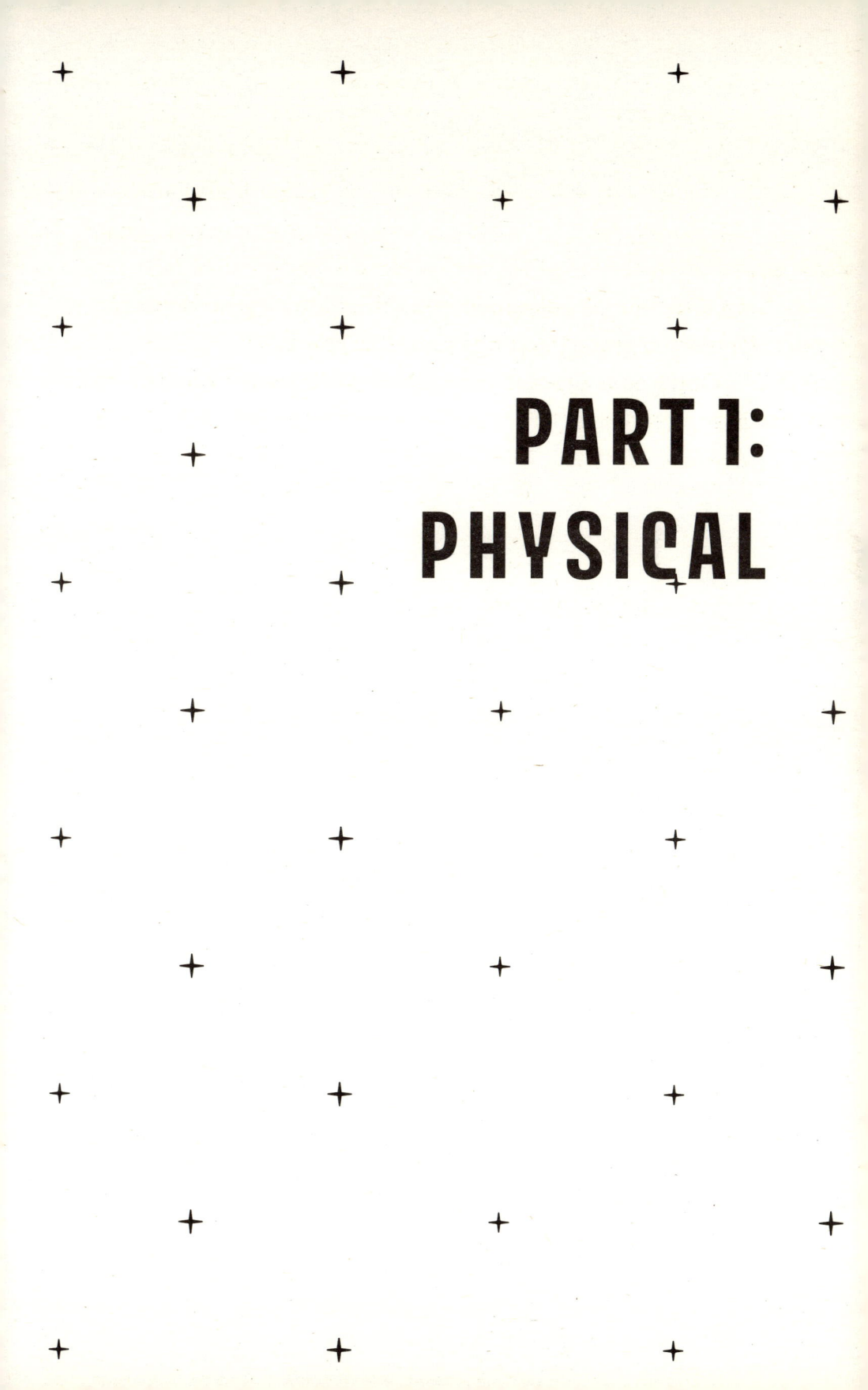

2

RESETTING YOUR RHYTHM

Quite a lot of attention is paid to the psychological reasons why people have problems with sleep, like stress, burnout and anxiety. These are important to address, but first I want you to focus on the physiology of sleep and how vital it is for you to be physically comfortable to welcome the sleep process. That's crucial.

In this chapter, there are four Sleep Hacks you can choose from. There are two other chapters dedicated to the Physical Sleep Hacks, so remember, you just need to pick one of the six Sleep Hacks in total from this section, to be combined with two from the other sections, Psychological and Hypnomagical.

MY PERSONAL SLEEP JOURNEY

My experience of sleep shows how your sleep patterns can change over your lifetime. These days I enjoy excellent sleep, and as I will show you, you can too. But I haven't always. Truth be told, it wasn't until I had a car accident in 2007 that I understood how strongly physiology and sleep are linked.

Earlier in my life, I used to sleep very little, but that was by choice. I had this mantra in my head, which I got from my dad: 'sleep when I'm dead'. In hindsight, I know that is the wrong attitude (sorry, Dad!), but in my late teens and early twenties, that's what I believed. I thought I was thriving on five hours' sleep and I believed I was being super-productive. Now I know that certainly wasn't the case and by following the mantra I was simply bringing the 'death' sleep sooner than fate would otherwise have decided for me. Sure, I was doing TV shows and enjoying success, but if I had been getting the optimal levels of sleep, my work would certainly have been better. My health would also have been better; at the time I was struggling with digestive problems and weight issues. Not getting enough sleep also affected my attitude. I always try to maintain a positive outlook, but if something went wrong in work or in life I was sometimes crankier than I needed to be. The noughties is the decade that I can pinpoint in my head where I was so busy being busy that sleep simply wasn't important to me. I started my TV career in 2003, with my first TV show, *Close Encounters with Keith Barry*, on RTÉ. The next year, I did my MTV show, *Brainwashed*, and in 2006 I began my CBS show in the US, *Keith Barry: Extraordinary*.

In 2008, I heard an interview with Will Smith. He was 39 at the time, and he'd already had huge success, not only as a rapper but also on TV in *The Fresh Prince of Bel-Air*, and then as a big movie star. In the interview on CBS News, he was asked what the secret of his success was. He said, 'I've never really viewed myself as particularly talented. I've viewed myself as slightly above average in talent. And where I excel is ridiculous, sickening work ethic. You know, while the other guy's sleeping? I'm working.' That resonated with me. In my head, from then on, from my twenties to mid-thirties, I told myself that when all the other magicians, hypnotists and mentalists are in bed, I'm out-working them. That's a flaw. For many years, I thought it was an amazing attribute, and I still do think that out-working everyone is a smart idea, but not to the detriment of sleep.

In the moment I thought I was doing amazing work, but when I look back now, while some of it I think was good and because I'm my own worst critic, some of it I think could have been so much better. What would have happened if I had got more sleep? Would my work have been better? The answer is a definitive yes.

What changed my attitude to sleep was the aftermath of a car accident. In March 2007, a car I was travelling in collided with another, head on, both doing around 60 miles per hour. I broke my knee; I had multiple fractures in my fibula and tibia; and my metatarsals (the bones going to your toes) were broken. My ankle was dislocated and my foot was wrapped around my shin, pointing the wrong way. The trauma surgeon in Daisy Hill Hospital in Co. Armagh spent 30 or 40 minutes trying to pull my foot back into place, to no avail – I was tensing my body so much it kept popping back out. Suddenly he stopped trying and said 'Keith, if you don't somehow relax your body, I'll need to amputate your foot.'

That was when everything shifted. I realised I needed to use all the hypnosis and brain-hacking techniques I had used on other people on myself. This sounds crazy, but right there and then I self-hypnotised myself into a deeply relaxed state of mind. Immediately the surgeon jolted my foot back into position and the nurse wrapped my whole leg and foot in an open leg cast. Ultimately, over three-and-a-half weeks, my leg had to be rebuilt up in the Royal Victoria Hospital in Belfast. After that, I struggled with my sleep because of the pain, especially in my ankle, which now has arthritis. Since the accident, I've also had problems with my back and shoulders and other areas of my body.

Pain is something we must all deal with. But the point is that even a minor ache or pain can keep you awake at night.

What I have uncovered, through the trials and tribulations that I've had since the car accident in 2007, is that the first step in getting good sleep is about relaxing your physical body and your whole physiology, which I'll explain to you how to do in a later chapter.

HOW GETTING MORE SLEEP IMPROVED MY LIFE

Before that, I want to let you know about how my wellbeing improved once I began to get more and better sleep.

MY ENERGY LEVELS SHOT UP

People often ask me, 'Where do you get your energy from?' There are two things I can put my energy down to. The first is that my internal purpose/my 'why' is clearly defined. That means I know exactly why I'm doing whatever I'm doing every day and what my future reality looks like. The second is sleep. I'm bouncing out of bed every morning because I've had restful, good sleep; I'm ready to attack the day. I'm definitely more productive and I'm managing to juggle a lot of projects quite well. I'm more focused than I've ever been. I have more projects going on than I've ever had in the past and I'm able to compartmentalise and focus on each and every one of them when I need to. If I'm focused on my family, I'm with them and I'm fully absorbed. When I'm on stage, I'm present with the audience and focused on them. While writing this book, I have been fully focused on that. If you don't have an optimal amount of sleep you can't function like that and you can't operate at the highest level.

MY RECOVERY FROM INJURY HAS IMPROVED

The link between recovery from injuries and getting enough sleep has been well documented.[3] There are several reasons why this is the case. The first is that in the deeper stages of sleep there's increased blood flow to the muscles, which allows oxygen and nutrients to regenerate cells. Another is that the hormone prolactin is released when you sleep, and this helps regulate inflammation. When I was in constant pain, my body was inflamed. I did various things to help this, including a breathing technique called the Wim Hof system, and an anti-inflammatory diet. But it wasn't until I addressed my sleep issues that the pain level truly went down. I found the pain getting less and less and I've been able to hit the gym hard every day and play football in the garden with my 12-year-old son, neither of which I had been able to do before.

There were other clear benefits too.

I'M ENJOYING PERFORMING ON STAGE A LOT MORE

When I wasn't getting enough sleep, I would get more nervous going on stage. I might mess up a demonstration or fail to hack someone's mind, sometimes in front of 1,500 people! Can you imagine the embarrassment? The stress was unimaginable.

I'M LESS CRANKY

Like many parents, I found myself getting short with my children and raising my voice with them when I shouldn't have, and I no longer do that. I find that I have way more patience with them, am more attentive to their needs, and have more fun moments with them every day.

And now let's turn to what you need to do to enjoy restorative, relaxing and regenerative sleep.

KNOW YOUR CIRCADIAN RHYTHMS

If you've read anything at all about the science of sleep, you'll have heard of circadian rhythms. These rhythms are a core part of our physiology, the 24-hour internal clock that includes a variety of processes including sleep–wake cycles, activity–rest cycles and eating–fasting cycles. Circadian rhythms mainly respond to light and dark, and they affect most living things, including animals, plants and microbes. It's so important to grasp the fact that we need to regulate these rhythms to optimise sleep, as well as our overall health and productivity.

The big issue is that, right now, more than at any other time in history, these rhythms are all over the place, largely because we're staring at screens and our smartphone is never out of our hands. Understanding that we are all tech addicts is a first step to solving our sleep issues. Light exposure is what keeps us alert during daytime, and natural sunlight is rich in blue spectrum light. But with so much artificial light coming at us via devices, computers and LED lights, it's confusing our bodies as to when we should go to sleep. If you're trying to limit your exposure to blue light – as you should – a recent analysis that looked at 17 studies from 6 different countries indicated that blue light blocking glasses do not work. This analysis found that adding a blue light filter to your glasses won't protect your eyes from strain, and it won't improve the quality of your sleep.

The other science aspect to be aware of is your brainwaves. These rhythmic patterns of neural activity are measured in hertz, and different waves are associated with different states. When you're awake, your brainwaves are in beta mode (12–38Hz). This is when you're focused, when you're problem-solving and when you're going about your everyday business. Alpha brainwaves (8–12Hz) happen when you're thinking quietly and you're relaxed, in almost a meditative state. Theta brainwaves (4–8Hz) are slower still. These waves are associated with daydreaming and feeling drowsy. You're not fully asleep, but perhaps thoughts from the day and thoughts about tomorrow are flitting in and out of your mind. It's a weird, dreamy state. Delta brainwaves (1–4Hz) are the slowest. I would love everyone reading this book to achieve delta brainwave sleep. This is slow wave sleep, the deepest stage of your sleep cycle, when you are most relaxed. Delta brainwave sleep has been described as the time when your body shuts down for repairs, and its many health benefits include greater immunity and longevity, and a reduction in inflammation and pain.

SLEEP HACK 1
TAKE IT OUTSIDE

The very first step in resetting your rhythm begins when you get up in the morning. I want you to build in this very important habit: go outside and get some low-level, natural sunlight into your eyes (indirectly, of course – never stare directly at the sun) for five to ten minutes.

All the current research indicates that morning sunlight regulates your circadian rhythm. Sunlight sends a signal to the brain that it's time to wake up, resulting in a decrease in the production of melatonin (the sleep hormone), and an increase in the stress hormone cortisol (an optimum level being necessary for wellbeing) and the feel-good neurotransmitter serotonin. The pineal gland metabolises serotonin into melatonin, which helps you naturally fall asleep at night.

Simply put, the sleep hormone melatonin is made from serotonin and people are often surprised when they learn this! If you don't have enough serotonin in your body, you won't make enough of the melatonin that is so necessary to achieve great sleep. In the next chapter, I'll be explaining more about how you can feed your brain and optimise serotonin levels, which can help your body produce melatonin.

Your pineal gland is located deep in your brain and its primary function is to regulate your circadian rhythms of sleep and wakefulness by secreting melatonin. Serotonin, which is derived from the amino acid tryptophan, is synthesised into melatonin in the pineal gland. This synthesis and secretion of melatonin is dramatically affected by the eyes' exposure to light: during daylight hours, concentrations of melatonin are low and they peak when it's dark.

I know you may be tempted to skip over this, but stop for a moment right now. Decide how important sleep is to you. Ask yourself this question: Am I willing to walk outside, even in the rain, to hear the birds sing, listen to the morning traffic, and say to myself 'It's a great day to be alive'? Or would I rather suffer tiredness, brain fog, and whatever other ailments may come down the line from lack of sleep? I suggest you think long and hard about this, as those five to ten minutes outside first thing in the morning could change your life for ever.

Andrew D. Huberman, associate professor of neurobiology at Stanford University School of Medicine, considers viewing morning sunlight among the top five of all actions that support mental health, physical health and performance. He advises that even on overcast days, there is still enough sunlight to have positive effects on your wellbeing, although you may have to increase the time outside to 15–20 minutes. If it's dark when you're getting up, he suggests turning on as many bright indoor artificial lights as possible, then getting outside as soon as the sun rises.

I know that the dark mornings may be when you struggle with this new habit of going outside first thing in the morning. I also know that the rain, cold and snow may deter you. Don't worry, I have a hack for you. I would suggest using a light therapy lamp, if you have access to one, on those dark mornings. These are also great if you're affected by seasonal affective disorder (SAD). The key is to get one that offers 10,000 lux of light exposure so that it has the same effect that sunlight has.

SLEEP HACK 2
ELIMINATE BAD HABITS

If you've had problems with your sleep, you are more than likely aware of some of the things you shouldn't be doing that might be interfering with the pursuit of a good night's shut-eye. Essentially, be sensible with your caffeine intake; and don't use electronic devices too close to bedtime. Here's a little refresh for you.

CUT THE CAFFEINE

Let's start with your caffeine intake. If you're serious about improving your sleep – and if you're reading this book, you clearly are – you have to look to your caffeine consumption. That can be tea, coffee, cola and energy drinks. Don't get me wrong, I love my coffee. But I also know that in a healthy person, the half-life of coffee (the time it takes for the starting amount of the substance to reduce by half in the body) is about five hours; but it can range from 1.5 to 9.5 hours depending on an individual's metabolism. This means that if I want to get deep sleep, and I'm planning to go to bed at 11 p.m., I'll have my last cup of coffee in the early afternoon. As a general rule of thumb, my cut-off point for coffee is lunchtime, unless I plan on staying up late. So enjoy your caffeinated drinks, but have them early in the day and don't have too many.

BANISH THE BLUE LIGHT

We've already touched on the second major bad habit that you need to eliminate. In these days of digitisation, we need to get to grips with the fact that our circadian rhythms are knocked all over the place a lot of the time because of the light entering our eyes, and specifically blue light. So you should put the phone down before you go to bed at night, and you should stop watching TV or using your laptop for at least an hour before you go to bed.

This is a very modern dilemma, and I look back to my grandfather as an example of how things have changed. He was a gardener and a handyman, and he worked hard outside all day. Then he'd come home and play cards at 5 p.m., followed by dinner and bed. I remember him always telling my sister and me what a great sleeper he was and how soundly he slept. Why did he sleep so well? Because that generation didn't spend their lives glued to a screen.

The blue light from phones, iPads, laptops and other devices interferes with sleep. This is so important I'm going to repeat it. You need to put the phone down before you go to bed, and you need to stop watching TV and stop using your laptop for at least an hour before you go to bed. This needs to become one of your 'immoveables' or what I call a non-negotiable.

A non-negotiable means that once you decide on a new habit you simply refuse to negotiate with yourself. For example, deciding that I will not use my phone in the morning until I've had at least five minutes outside has become a gamechanger for me. Not only am I sleeping better but my overall mood and productivity have improved.

Some people say that you need to get the phone out of the bedroom entirely. I don't subscribe to that, as I like to have it in the room in case of an emergency. What I do is put my phone on airplane mode, face down on the bedside table, so that's there no light coming out of it. Then I just don't touch it again. If you think you might be tempted to have a sneaky look on your phone and then 15 minutes later you've gone down a rabbit hole, do get your phone out of the room. 'But I need my phone for the alarm,' people say. I say: buy a cheap analogue alarm clock. Worried that the alarm clock won't go off? Buy two. I find that when I'm abroad on business I really can't sleep at all for fear of not waking up for an early morning flight. I'm wondering if my smartphone alarm will go off or not. To fix that I bought two super-cheap analogue alarm clocks that travel around the world with me. I'm not relying on my smartphone for the alarm and I'm confident that at least one of the analogue alarms will work. That single habit has helped me more than anything else to sleep deeply when I'm travelling. At a more extreme level, you can even buy a lockbox with a self-controlled timer for your smartphone. But before you take a drastic step like that, if you are struggling with not looking at your phone in bed or before bed, I'd like you to try my Swipe strategy to break this bad habit.

TRY THIS: THE SWIPE TECHNIQUE In order to break your phone habit, we have to break it down subconsciously. This is a quick neuro-linguistic programming (NLP) brain hack you can do in the evening; it shouldn't take up more than two minutes of your time and it's a very useful tool to help you achieve the discipline necessary to put the phone down. Remember, the smartphone completely undermines sleep quality.

- Sit or lie down in a safe, comfortable place.
- Close your eyes and imagine your smartphone is as tall and wide as a skyscraper.
- On that giant smartphone, in your mind's eye, visualise yourself in bed on your smartphone, as your cortisol and serotonin levels increase, causing you to feel wide awake.
- See yourself having a disturbed night's sleep because of this bad habit. Fast forward to the next morning where you are groggy, tired and lethargic. Decide immediately this is not the future you want or desire.
- Now pause that picture, drain it of its colour, and swipe left with a new image appearing in its place.
- Visualise this image being you taking the phone, putting it on airplane mode, and immediately putting it down as you prepare for the restful night's sleep ahead. See yourself sleeping soundly all night long.

> Fast forward to the next morning where you notice you are now alert, full of energy and ready to attack the day with positivity and determination.
> Next, swipe left again and see the words: 'My new non-negotiable is "no phone in bed"' appearing on the giant smartphone inside your mind.
> Open your eyes and continue about your day.

You can do this technique for as long as is required until you break your phone habit – for some people, it could be once, others 10 times, and it might be longer for others. Commit to this NLP brain hack until you find yourself putting the phone away each and every time you head to bed.

So what do you do in the hour before bed if you're not on your phone or watching Netflix? You could chat with your loved one, or your family. If you're alone, you could start your to-do list, more of which a bit later.

E-readers are not an option, as research has shown that the light emitted from e-readers suppresses melatonin.[4] But I do recommend reading an actual physical book before bed – provided it's not too exciting with a plot that will keep you awake. Reading before bed is a known de-stresser – there's a reason why a bedtime story is part of most children's bedtime routine.

As a hypnotist, something I often do is anchor thoughts in people and then trigger those thoughts. During a show, I might hypnotise someone and tell them that in a few moments they're going to wake up and genuinely believe that they're an alien from

Mars. I get them to open their eyes, ask them their name and just start chatting. It's only when I touch them on the shoulder that the anchor is triggered and they'll start talking gibberish, or 'Martian'. But here's the interesting thing: I can now build on that anchor. I can tell this same person that the next time I tap them on the shoulder they're going to believe they are Elvis, and whatever their belief system or their gender, that's who they'll become.

You can use the anchor-trigger effect to build new and healthier habits for sleep. You simply decide on a healthy anchor, and that in turn triggers the next one. For example, you're sitting down watching your favourite TV show in the evening alone or with your partner. Now create an anchor that when the TV show is over, the phone is turned off, as well as all electronic devices. This could then trigger you into writing your to-do list, and next you're triggered to practise the Swipe technique, and so on.

SLEEP HACK 3
MAKE YOUR BEDROOM SLEEP-FRIENDLY

You have to make a decision about your bedroom. That decision is to only use your bedroom for the three S's: sleep, sex and sickness. Nothing else. Because of remote working, a lot of people are using their bedroom as a home office. That needs to stop. Even if you have a small home or a busy household, find another room to work in.

IT'S ALL ABOUT THE TEMPERATURE

The number one thing for me when it comes to making a bedroom sleep-friendly is the temperature. Studies have shown that the optimal temperature for sleep is 19–21°C.[5] Many people like to set up a warm, cosy bed, but this will actually interfere with getting a good night's sleep. In the lead-up to bed, your body temperature drops, as a way of preparing you for sleep. It's one of the reasons why vigorous exercise before bed isn't a good idea. Keep your bedroom cool. During winter, turn off the radiator in the bedroom and let the natural heat of the house warm it up. In summer, if you can and it's not a security issue, crack open the window for a couple of hours before bedtime.

LET THERE BE (LOW) LIGHT

I also want to start tricking my system immediately in preparation for sleep when I enter the bedroom, and this means low-level light. Obviously if you have a dimmer light in your bedroom, that's a great way to make it sleep-friendly. I don't have dimmer lights but I do have a low-wattage light bulb – 40 watts. It's enough to see your way to the bathroom if you need to get up in the night but it's not too bright, and it doesn't stop melatonin being naturally released into the body. I use a low-light reading light when I'm journaling or reading in bed.

CONSIDER BETTER BEDDING

It's important to me that buying this book is the main investment you need to make to improve your sleep. I'm not going to suggest you have to buy 1,000-thread sheets or a mega-expensive mattress, but if you are replacing anything in your bedroom, I can give you some guidelines.

Lots of people have a bad mattress – it might be saggy or uncomfortable. If you're not in the market for a new one, a mattress topper is a fairly inexpensive way of making your bed more sleep-friendly.

Pillows are crucial, and I've tried them all. Find ones that are comfortable, that support your head and neck, and that keep your shoulders, hips and spine in alignment. A lot of people swear by buckwheat pillows, which are natural, organic and a good alternative to synthetic varieties, but they're also quite pricey. I have to be honest and say that buckwheat pillows were not for me, but they do provide excellent support because they mould to the shape of your head and neck.

Bed linen is also key. I recommend sleeping under a light sheet in summer and a light duvet when it's colder. They have to be comfortable, the most comfortable you can afford. If you have bed linen that's starchy and cardboard-like around the body, it's not going to help induce a good night's sleep.

WEAR SOMETHING COMFY

The same goes for what you wear to bed, if you do wear anything. Again, comfort is king: don't buy something because you think it looks great or because you like the colour. Pyjamas, or similar, don't need to be expensive; they just need to be comfy and ideally made from natural fibres that help regulate body temperature. Here's a clothing hack not many people know for those hot summer nights. Freeze your pyjamas. Well, not completely! Put them in an airtight bag in the freezer for 30 minutes before bedtime. I love doing this during the summer and now have the whole family doing it to help cool down in preparation for a good night's sleep.

Something else that is in my sleep arsenal is a blindfold or sleep mask. As a mentalist I've had blindfolds in my hand since I was 14 years old and I perform a lot of demonstrations with them. You could say I know them inside out. I think I've found the best one for sleep, a brand called Mzoo, which you can get online. I like it because its hollow design prevents my eyes and eyelids coming into contact with the blindfold, and it puts me into complete darkness. But if you don't want to invest in a blindfold, having something to hand that you can grab and throw over your eyes, like a T-shirt or scarf, also works. Blindfolds – or some variation – are really useful if you share a bed with someone who gets up in the night and turns on the lights.

TRY THIS: CREATE DARKNESS IN YOUR BEDROOM Use some black electrical tape to block out any small LED indicator lights or appliance lights in your bedroom to help create darkness.

MANAGE YOUR SLEEP PARTNER

Which leads me to: what do you do if you have a disruptive partner who always gets up in the night or who snores? Snoring is easy to resolve – get yourself a pair of earplugs. I'm not a fan of separate bedrooms for couples, as I don't think it's good for relationships, but if you need to, and have another bedroom to do so, you can try that route. For the partner who gets up in the night, disturbing you, it's about having an open and honest conversation with them. Say 'I need you to do me a favour. If you're getting up in the night, please do it quietly without banging around. My sleep is so important and it affects my mood, my productivity and health. I know you understand how important sleep is to me.'

Or you can stop reading now, hand them the book and tell them to read the following lines from me to them:

'Hey, you. Yes, you. Keith Barry here. *Stop* banging around in the middle of the night and understand that your partner who is reading this understands the importance of sleep and needs your help to rest deeply at night. Thanks!'

However, if someone is in a deep delta brainwave sleep, they shouldn't be woken up by their partner, as long as that partner is relatively quiet.

PUT SOME MUSIC ON

Another thing to try to make your bedroom sleep-friendly is gentle music. There are several studies that suggest that music helps sleep because it regulates hormones and triggers the release of dopamine, a feel-good hormone which helps address pain. Relaxing music helps slow down your heart and your brainwaves, and it helps to relieve anxiety, which may be preventing you getting to sleep. Studies indicate that music improves sleep quality by reducing sympathetic nervous system activity and decreasing blood pressure and respiratory rate.[6]

SCENT YOUR SLEEPING SPACE

Pleasant smells, such as lavender, are associated with falling asleep easily, but it's not something I can stand behind with any authority. What I know about smell is only what I've read about it. I have no sense of smell (which doctors think might be genetic), so lighting an aromatherapy candle is not part of my sleep ritual. While it's not a magic cure, studies show that a scented candle can benefit sleep by reducing stress and triggering a relaxation response.

SLEEP HACK 4
DEVELOP A SLEEP ROUTINE

The reason for developing a sleep routine is to produce melatonin at night, which as I've already outlined, is necessary for sleep. I'm not going to be too prescriptive about this because everyone is different. My friend Al goes to bed at 9.30 p.m. but he gets up at 5.30 a.m. He'll text me and ask me if I want to go for a swim with him at 6 a.m., and I'll say no, I can't go for a swim at 6 a.m. because I'm going to be working until midnight. There are many people like me who don't have a set schedule; one night I might go to bed at 11 p.m., another night it might be 1 a.m. But even within those variations, you can have a routine where you still get your optimal amount of sleep. There are 10 steps in this sleep routine.

1. **Decide what time you are going to bed and what your wake-up time will be**
   Base this on your schedule and work backwards by seven hours or eight hours – you know what the optimal amount of sleep is for you to perform at your best. For example, if you need to be up at 6.30 a.m., you should start winding down before 11 p.m. The next step is:

2. **Write your to-do list for the following day**
   This is a great way to ease the mental load, reduce stress and prepare for the following day, as I mentioned in the previous chapter.

3. **Have a small glass of water or a warm, relaxing drink like chamomile or valerian root tea**

   Drinking fluids before bed can help with digestion and keep the body hydrated during sleep – although not too much, as you don't want to be woken by a call of nature in the middle of the night. Science backs the benefits of herbal beverages for sleep. According to the Sleep Foundation, after analysing 60 research studies researchers found that valerian root can likely improve sleep and reduce anxiety. There are lots of other sleep-promoting herbal teas on the market. Find one you like and make it part of your sleep routine.

4. **Call time on your devices**

   That's TV, computer, Kindle and phone all off at least one hour before you plan to go to bed. Use this time to chat with your housemates or family, clean the house, iron, write your to-do list or do any other activity that doesn't require a screen. Remember: no screens for one hour before bed. That is a non-negotiable.

5. **Practise the Swipe technique**

   Flick back to page 42 to remind yourself how to do this. Do it in any quiet room in the house before you enter the bedroom. Then put your phone away until the time you have decided you are going to pick it up again, which should be the next morning – but only after you have been outside in sunlight for a few minutes.

6. **Get into your night clothes**
   As discussed above, whatever you choose to wear in bed has to be comfortable. As a general rule, natural fibres are always better. If cold feet are an issue, try some socks and see if they help your sleep.

7. **Do your night-time cleansing ritual**
   This includes washing your teeth, cleaning your face and using any other lotions and potions that you like to use in preparation for bed.

8. **Get into bed and make sure you're as comfortable as possible**
   Make sure that the light is low-level, the bedclothes feel good, and you feel good.

9. **Read a (physical) book and/or listen to some relaxing music**
   Some really soothing music in the background as you're reading your book can be very beneficial. I'm not into classical music so I'll just put on some random instrumental music or binaural beats when I'm getting ready to go to sleep. Binaural beats are an illusion created by the brain when you listen to two tones with slightly different frequencies at the same time and they can help you enter a meditative state.

10. **Lights out**
    Get ready to drift off to sleep by using some of my visualisation techniques, which you'll find in the next part of the book

This sounds simple, and it is. Is it easy? You will have to commit yourself to this routine, but by ingraining it into your evening, you will soon start to see the benefits.

3

FEED YOUR BRAIN: EAT WELL TO SLEEP WELL

In his book *The Physiology of Taste*, published in 1825, lawyer, writer and early advocate of low-carb eating Jean Anthelme Brillat-Savarin famously wrote: 'Tell me what you eat and I will tell you what you are.' My riff on that is: 'Tell me what you eat and I will tell you how you sleep.' I see it a lot in my work as a mind coach with enormously successful people running massive companies who struggle with their sleep and wonder why, when they're living on a diet of processed foods, caffeine and energy drinks.

Picture this: Paddy is a successful business owner, with a thriving company raking in €6 million annually, surrounded by adoring friends and family who marvel at his achievements. To all outward appearances, he had it all. But beneath the surface, a storm was brewing.

As I sat across from him, I could see the weariness etched on his face. He looked like a man who had been drained of his vitality, his energy sapped by an invisible force. And there, on his chest, a tell-tale sign of distress – a noticeable rash. I couldn't ignore the signs any longer; something was seriously amiss in his life. I decided to probe deeper, to uncover the root of his troubles. 'How is your sleep?' I asked, and his response was startlingly bleak. 'Non-existent,' he admitted. 'I manage to grab a few hours a night, but most nights I find myself on YouTube, watching mindless videos in the dead of night before drifting off again.'

My concern deepened as I delved further into his daily routine. 'What about your diet?' I asked. His answer was troubling: 'I start the day with a cup of coffee and a cigarette. I skip breakfast, but I have a hearty lunch around 2 p.m. – a chicken roll, loaded with butter, mayonnaise, lettuce, and chicken. Dinner consists of meat, a solitary vegetable, and some potatoes. And in between all of this, I'm smoking 40 cigarettes a day, washing it down with roughly six cups of coffee.'

It was a recipe for disaster, a relentless onslaught on his body's wellbeing. Instead of focusing on time management and non-verbal communication (which is what he had hired me to teach him), I knew I had to pivot, and fast, like a magician invisibly switching cards under the nose of a spectator in a millisecond. This wasn't about business any more; this was about saving a life.

I made it abundantly clear to him that no level of success was worth subjecting his body to such extreme stress. The intertwined issues of sleep deprivation and poor nutrition were like the intertwined elements of a bird's nest – twigs, leaves, and feathers, all interconnected. The rash that had spread across his body was merely a symptom of a much deeper problem – his hormones were out of balance, his body screaming for help.

You might think his case is an extreme one, but I challenge you to look within yourself. Maybe you don't smoke 40 cigarettes a day, but do you have a vice of your own? Perhaps a couple of cigarettes, a few too many vapes, or an excess of coffee? And what about your meals? Are they truly nourishing your body and aiding in its repair?

The advice I offered him, in that critical moment, is the same advice I'm sharing with you now.

Food works as a very powerful agent in relation to your sleep. I pay attention to what I eat, for a variety of reasons. As I've mentioned, I have acquired several injuries over the years and I have found that an anti-inflammation diet helps with that. I also take note of what I eat because my schedule is fairly hectic and I'm constantly travelling for work. So that I can give it my all and have sufficient energy reserves to get everything I need to do done, perform at my optimal levels, and still be fully focused on my family when I'm with them, I'm mindful of my diet, but not unhealthily obsessed with it. What I've also learned over the years is that both the type of food I eat and when I eat it have a significant impact on the quality of my sleep.

As a side note, I have also practised intermittent fasting on and off for years. Simply put, it's when you don't eat for a specific time frame, and there are lots of ways you can do it. A fast generally lasts from 12 to 24 hours, but I am a fan of the 14:10 method. That means going 14 hours with no food (this includes your sleeping hours) and eating within a 10-hour window. It's been proven to help with inflammation, which is why I began doing it, but it's also been shown to benefit sleep by reinforcing your circadian rhythms.[7]

I'd like to introduce to you a whole range of foods that can improve your sleep, and which have been scientifically proven to do so. While I have a first-class chemistry degree, I left the world of science behind to pursue my dream of being a magician, hypnotherapist and brain hacker; but I still have a good understanding of the science behind the claims for these foods, and it's all solid. Of course, if you are planning any radical changes to your diet, you should always chat to your GP first and check that it's okay.

In the last chapter, I talked about melatonin, what it is and how it works. Quick recap: it's the sleep hormone, which we want our bodies to produce lots of at night-time, and it's metabolised from serotonin, the feel-good neurotransmitter that regulates mood, helps you think and wakes you up in the morning. We also want our bodies to produce lots of this. In the US and other parts of the world, melatonin is classed as a food supplement, so you can buy it at health food stores. It's popular with frequent flyers because these tablets can reduce or even prevent jetlag. In Ireland, this shortcut to sleep isn't available over the counter. The Health Products Regulatory Authority (HPRA), which regulates medicines in Ireland, classes it as a medicine. You can get it on prescription – it's called Circadin – and it's generally prescribed to people over 55 to help with short-term sleep problems. It's the same situation in the UK.

Given the amount of time we spend on screens, it's not surprising that our melatonin levels could do with a helping hand. The good news is you don't need to buy a bottle of pills in order to naturally encourage the production of melatonin in your pineal gland. What

I'd like you to do is to start eating more natural foods that will promote melatonin production and also serotonin production.

There's no magic bullet when it comes to food that can improve your sleep cycle. Health and sleep are strongly related, and if you're not coming from a good baseline, and your normal diet is takeaways, ultra-processed foods and zero fruit and veg, a handful of nuts isn't going to sort out your sleep issues. Looking at your diet is another non-negotiable, as is adding some of these foods to your meals every day.

SLEEP HACK 5
CHOOSE TWO FOOD ITEMS TO EAT EACH DAY FROM THIS LIST

THE FOLLOWING IS A SELECTION OF FOODS THAT HAVE BEEN SCIENTIFICALLY PROVEN TO POTENTIALLY AID SLEEP:

- Cherries
- Walnuts
- Almonds
- Pecans
- Oats
- Bananas
- Kiwis
- Spinach
- Live yoghurt
- Turkey
- Salmon or other oily fish
- Passion fruit
- Dragon fruit

- Pumpkin seeds
- Cheese
- Prunes
- Wholegrains
- Watermelon

Have a read through the following before deciding which you would like to incorporate into your daily diet.

CHERRIES

It doesn't get more delicious than chowing down on a handful of fresh cherries. The fact that they can help with sleep is an added bonus. The reason why they're a sleep aid is that cherries contain small amounts of melatonin, as well as tryptophan, an amino acid that is used to make both melatonin and serotonin. They also contain vitamin A, vitamin C and magnesium, making them a nutritional powerhouse of a fruit. Magnesium also promotes sleep, and I'll get into that presently. Cherries not in season, or not in your local supermarket? Cherry juice will also do the trick; one study showed that cherry juice had a beneficial effect on sleep in older adults with insomnia.[8] There is a caveat, though: the cherries or the cherry juice must be tart. Naturally sour cherries like the Montmorency variety, which has high levels of phytochemicals, including melatonin, are a great source of melatonin. Studies have indicated that tart cherries can be beneficial in improving sleep duration and quality in healthy men and women and might also help manage disturbed sleep.[9]

WALNUTS

Another all-natural way to eat your way to better sleep, walnuts – raw – are tasty, portable, handy snacks. They contain high levels of ALA, an anti-inflammatory omega-3 acid, which can benefit heart health, memory and skin, and help fight inflammation. Crucially when it comes to sleep, walnuts contain tryptophan, the amino acids that the body uses to produce serotonin and melatonin. Not only that, but walnuts also actually contain melatonin itself, the oh-so-important sleep hormone. Of all the nuts, walnuts have the highest melatonin content,[10] and it gets better. Walnuts also contain magnesium and can contribute to your overall daily intake. You may not be aware of this, but a huge number of people don't consume enough magnesium. It's a nutrient that is needed for so many things: the heart's electrical activity, skeletal muscle relaxation, nerve transmission and restful sleep, and that's only some of its functions. However, according to studies, magnesium deficiency is a common and under-recognised problem worldwide. It works in a different way from melatonin, which tells your body when it's time for sleep; magnesium can help quiet the nerves that might keep you awake because it plays a role in regulating GABA, a neurotransmitter that reduces a nerve cell's capacity to receive or send chemical messages to other nerve cells. Magnesium also calms down N-methyl-D-aspartate receptor, an excitable neurotransmitter in the brain. If you're not a fan of walnuts, or if you have a nut allergy, you can do as I do and get a magnesium spray. Although it's better to get your magnesium through your food, and there isn't enough research into how effective magnesium is when it's applied topically, I find it's very relaxing and it has certainly benefited my sleep – my wife also says it smells amazing.

ALMONDS

Another nut you should stock up on, and they should be in their raw form, not roasted or salted, although, if we're going get nerdy about it, almonds don't actually meet the botanical criteria to be classified as a nut. (And by the way, just to drive some of you crazy, I pronounce the 'l' in almonds!) Technically, they're what are known as drupes, or seeds, because they grow inside a fleshy fruit and have to be shelled before they can be eaten. A true nut is the fruit of the tree that dries and hardens, like chestnuts and hazelnuts – remember this the next time you're doing a table quiz. Almonds have many of the same sleep-beneficial properties as walnuts. They're a natural and rich source of melatonin and they also have lots of the other 'm' we want when we're trying to improve our sleep: magnesium. About 28g of raw almonds – approximately 23 nuts – will give you approximately 18 per cent of your recommended magnesium for the day. Almonds also contain small amounts of the amino acid tryptophan, which as I've already mentioned is the precursor to serotonin and melatonin. As a snack, they have lots of other good nutrients to recommend them, like vitamin E, phosphorous, riboflavin and fibre.

PECANS

These are also great, and I like to have them to hand to snack on. They contain melatonin, magnesium, zinc, vitamin B1 and lots of other good things.

OATS

You're probably thinking oats are more of a breakfast thing, and I agree, oats are an excellent start to the day. But they are also a good evening snack. If you're concerned about oatmeal being too carby, and causing a blood sugar spike, rest assured that this isn't the case. Because they're so rich in fibre, oats provide slow-release energy, meaning that your blood sugar levels won't go crazy. Oats also contain excellent amounts of those two magic ingredients, melatonin and magnesium. They also have plenty of tryptophan, the amino acid that's also a sleep superstar. The easiest way to eat oats is to make a jar of overnight oats, which will last in the fridge for up to four days. This is a no-cook method – you leave the oats to soak overnight in water and/or milk (or a dairy-free alternative), and you can then add other ingredients like seeds, nuts and fruit. You'll find lots of recipes online. It's creamy and delicious and, nutritionally speaking, overnight soaked oats have more fibre than cooked oats.

BANANAS

We love our bananas in Ireland. In fact, we import more of them than any other fruit, so there's no reason why you shouldn't add them to your shopping basket. Bananas have been called 'nature's sleeping pill' and one of the reasons why eating them can help improve the quality of your sleep is because they contain tryptophan. They also have vitamin B6, which helps tryptophan produce the sleep hormone melatonin. Added to that, bananas are a great source of magnesium, and one banana will give you 8 per cent of your daily magnesium requirements. Bananas are also an excellent source of potassium, which will help calm your muscles at night. I like to just eat them raw, or whizz them up in a smoothie.

KIWIS

These are amazing and they're no chore to eat. Rich in serotonin, the brain chemical that regulates our sleep cycle, kiwis are strongly linked with better sleep. One study from 2011 found that eating kiwis on a daily basis made dramatic improvements to sleep, with the kiwi-eating participants falling asleep more quickly, sleeping more soundly, having better quality sleep and sleeping more overall.[11] Another recent study found that consumption of two kiwis one hour before bed for four weeks has the potential to positively impact the sleep and recovery of elite athletes.[12]

SPINACH

Eat your greens, we were always told as kids, and of course it's good advice. Spinach is a very nutritious vegetable to pile onto your plate at your evening meal. Some of its sleep-friendly nutrients include magnesium to regulate melatonin and vitamin B9, which helps regulate the production of serotonin. If you're not keen on spinach, try kale, which is another leafy green packed with magnesium, to calm the body and encourage sleep.

LIVE YOGHURT

Live yoghurt is yoghurt that has been fermented with gut-friendly bacteria. If you don't have a problem with dairy, you should be adding this to your diet because a healthy gut helps with sleep, and proper sleep benefits your gut. Other research has shown that poor sleep can lead to imbalances in the gut microbiota, reducing the number of good bacteria and potentially promoting the growth of harmful ones.[13] We should be doing all we can to look after our gut health, and eating live yoghurt is a good way of doing that, as it's also associated with healthier dietary patterns, reduced weight and an increase in good bacteria in the gut.[14]

TURKEY

Turkey makes you tired; you've probably experienced yourself when you've had a snooze after a massive Christmas dinner. But in truth that's more likely to do with all the carbs that you've consumed, rather than the turkey itself. Turkey (and chicken) is a rich source of tryptophan, which the body doesn't make and which is the precursor to serotonin and is also needed to synthesise melatonin. You can incorporate turkey slices into your breakfast (one study showed that eating a tryptophan-rich breakfast, combined with exposure to sunlight, increased melatonin production at night.[15] Or make turkey or chicken your protein choice for your evening meal. For vegetarians, tofu is a great source of tryptophan.

SALMON

Or, indeed, any other oily fish. A research study found that people who ate salmon three times a week over a period of months had better overall sleep. The reason behind this is because fatty fish contain vitamin D and omega-3 fatty acids, which help regulate serotonin. Another study from the University of Oxford, which focused on children who had sleep issues, found that the children got 58 more minutes of sleep at night, and also had fewer waking issues, after being given DHA, the omega-3 acid found in oily fish, krill oil and algae oil.[16]

The kind of salmon you should eat is wild Atlantic salmon. Farmed salmon is pumped full of red dye to make it look like wild salmon, and it can also contain antibiotics. Always go wild when it comes to salmon.

Fish oils are key. I take cod liver oil every morning, not just for my joints but also to feed my brain and help it work properly. If you're eating oily fish several times a week, you probably don't need a fish oil supplement. If you're not, it's something to consider, not just for your sleep but for your overall wellbeing. If you're vegan or vegetarian, seaweed and algae supplements are available.

PASSION FRUIT

This is one of my favourite things to eat and it's regarded as a natural sedative. Passion fruit has several medicinal alkaloids, including harman, which has traditionally been used to treat anxiety, as well as fibre, niacin, phosphorus and vitamins A and C, all of which are needed for healthy body functions.

DRAGON FRUIT

What's this? you might ask. It's a tropical fruit, also known as a strawberry pear, that grows in Mexico and along the Pacific coast. It's another natural sedative, as it's high in magnesium and also contains the amino acid tryptophan, those known sleep aids. I eat dragon fruit several times a week. You might wonder where you can get passion fruit and dragon fruit. I order these fruits online, and they come direct from the country of source straight to my door. I use CrowdFarming, a conglomerate of fully certified organic farmers around Europe (www.crowdfarming.com), which means you deal directly with the farmer. It's a little more expensive than picking up your fruit in a supermarket but it's an option that's well worth considering if you're serious about your sleep and your diet.

PUMPKIN SEEDS

These are great to nibble on, tossed over salads or stirred into your overnight oats. Pumpkin seeds contain heaps of nutrients that can potentially improve your sleep. They're a good source of magnesium, the relaxing mineral; our favourite amino acids; tryptophan; and also zinc, which raises serotonin levels.

CHEESE

A controversial one, this, as we've been told that eating cheese at night gives rise to all sorts of vivid and frightening dreams. But there's no strong scientific evidence to back that up. The calcium in cheeses such as Swiss and Cheddar helps the brain use the tryptophan found in dairy to make melatonin. The National Sleep Foundation, a non-profit, charitable organisation in the US, recommends cottage cheese as an evening snack because of its high tryptophan content.

PRUNES

A highly under-rated addition to your sleep-friendly diet. Prunes are well known for their high fibre content and keeping you regular, but they also have magnesium, the sleep mineral. Aligned with that, prunes – which are just dried plums – contain vitamin B6 and calcium, which combine to make melatonin. They taste sweet but they won't cause a spike in blood sugar levels. If you don't like eating them as is, try using them to make sugar-free desserts, or use them as a topping on wholegrain toast in the mornings.

WHOLEGRAINS

You probably know that wholegrains are good for your overall health, but you may not know that they can also aid sleep. Quinoa, for example, contains lots of magnesium and tryptophan; brown rice contains GABA, which calms the nervous system; and rice, barley and oats are all natural sources of melatonin. Complex carbohydrates like these aren't highly processed and, as the National Sleep Foundation in the US notes, the carbohydrate helps deliver tryptophan to the brain.

WATERMELON
Not necessarily something you'd think would help with sleep, but watermelon is actually a good source of potassium and magnesium. It also contains fibre and as it's 80 per cent water; a bowl of chopped watermelon some hours before you go to bed should keep you hydrated throughout the night. One caveat, though: it can have a slightly diuretic effect, so don't eat it too close to bedtime, as you might need to get up to use the bathroom in the middle of the night.

I appreciate that not everybody will like all of these sleep-friendly foods. Some people have food intolerances or allergies, or they might choose not to eat a food for religious or ideological reasons. That's fine. But what I ask you to do is this:

Every week, decide on a food from the above list that you're going to eat every morning to promote the release of serotonin, and also a food that becomes part of your dinner that promotes the release of melatonin.

For example, commit to yourself that every morning you'll have a handful of walnuts with your breakfast, and that your dinner is going to include lean turkey or chicken. Or perhaps you'll choose to start with kiwis as part of your breakfast, and then for your last meal of the day you'll load up your plate with spinach alongside whatever else you're having. You can try different foods for the subsequent week and the next one. Commit to this and you're committing to optimising your sleep cycle.

CHOOSE YOUR FLUIDS WISELY

Staying hydrated is vital, but what you're drinking is equally important. I mentioned caffeine in the previous chapter, and I'm not saying that you should give up your caffeine hit, but it's important that you limit caffeine intake to the earlier part of the day.

Some people think it's okay to have a herbal tea just before they go to bed. I think herbal teas are wonderful – and the calming, soothing benefits of chamomile, valerian root and other herbal teas have been scientifically proven. But you need to drink it at least one hour before you go to bed, because no matter what you're consuming, it's still taxing the digestive system. A small glass of water closer to bedtime is fine, but not too large a glass, because otherwise you'll have to deal with a call of nature at 4 a.m.

Green tea is another drink I love. It is bursting with antioxidants, essential for overall wellbeing, and it also has the amino acid theanine, which promotes relaxation and reduces stress. A word to the wise, though; make sure you're drinking decaffeinated green tea because otherwise it's going to hinder and not help your sleep.

One of my favourite things to drink in the morning is a lump of natural fresh ginger, half a lemon with the rind peeled off and a good bit of the pulp left on for fibre. Then I'll put three shakes of pink Himalayan salt onto the lemon and half a teaspoon of turmeric, add water and put it into my blender, and what I get is an anti-inflammatory glass of goodness. It starts the digestive process in an easy way for anyone who, like me, suffers from acid reflux.

There's also widespread interest in nutrition circles about adding pink Himalayan salt to water ('sole water'), and whether it can help people's digestion. There haven't been enough studies done to conclusively prove its health benefits, but I am a fan, as I do know pink Himalayan salt contains up to 84 minerals.

And now a little bit about alcohol. It negatively affects your sleep cycle and that's a fact. It may feel as though it gives you a deep sleep, but it's not a restful sleep. I know some people might say, 'But I have two glasses of red wine for my cardiovascular health, and it's not affecting my sleep.' However, they're wrong. I could cite so many studies that have proved categorically that alcohol is really terrible for sleep. But I don't want to sound preachy. I've made an agreement with myself that, potentially, alcohol might knock two years off my life. I might end up living to 76 and not 78 if I choose to drink alcohol in moderation throughout my life. I'm okay with that, and that's my choice. I drink alcohol but I limit my intake and make sure it's just at the weekends. But it doesn't detract from the hard, cold proof that if you have a drink every night in a week, your body is not going to rest and repair. In a nutshell, having too much alcohol regularly is associated with chronic sleep disturbances, lower delta wave sleep and more rapid eye movement sleep. Yes, you might fall asleep quicker when you've had a few drinks, but the quality of sleep you are getting is extremely poor. So now that you have the facts, it's your call on how committed you are to improving your sleep and if you want to eliminate alcohol from the equation and see if your sleep improves.

WHAT I EAT IN A DAY

Life is busy, busy, busy. But I'm still mindful of my sleep and therefore I'm mindful of what I eat. I'll give you an example of what I eat on the days I'm in full control of my schedule. This is what I eat in an ideal scenario (obviously not on a day when I'm intermittent fasting), but that doesn't mean I hit this every day – we all have bad days, and I'm not trying to put myself on any kind of pedestal.

In the morning, I'll get up and have my turmeric/ginger/lemon/pink Himalayan salt mix drink. Sometimes I'll throw some raw garlic in there, but that can be quite hard to stomach. I drink that first thing and then wait another half an hour to an hour before I eat.

My breakfast during the colder months is oats with berries – strawberries, blueberries. You might be wondering where I get these in winter, but I just use frozen berries if they're not seasonal. I'll also have a banana with that and of course my coffee.

During summer, one of my more unusual breakfasts is a banana omelette. I mash a banana in a bowl, add two egg whites, whisk it all together and then add in a scoop of chocolate whey protein powder. Now, I go to the gym a lot and I used to eat a lot of protein bars. But, truth be told, they're absolute rubbish, as they are packed with additives and highly processed. However, I do use a high-quality protein powder in my omelette and although it's processed it has minimal additives. This is a conscious choice to make sure I'm keeping my protein intake quite high. You don't have to put it in, but I do. For the omelette, I then melt ghee on the pan – it has a very low smoke point – and cook the omelette. Then I'll add goji berries – another superfood associated with improved sleep – and crumble some walnuts onto the omelette and have that with a side of berries. Sometimes I'll have a portion of fruit as well, like half a dragon fruit. It might seem like an odd start to the day, but this is a power breakfast: protein from the eggs and protein powder, carbs from the bananas and all the sleep-friendly nutrients in nuts.

After that, I'm generally out on the road. I'll have nuts in the car as a snack and usually an apple – I have apple trees in my garden, so, when they're in season, this is all organic. When I'm travelling any distance, I've learned to avoid the food in service stations. There is hardly any proper food in service stations – 90 per cent of it is just crisps and chocolates and doughnuts, etc., all ultra-processed. That's not to say we shouldn't ever eat these – we deserve a treat every once in a while. I don't pretend to live like a monk and don't want to come across like I do. But in preparation for getting good sleep that night, I'll have a Ziploc bag with a handful of walnuts, pecans and almonds in the car.

Lunch might be a chicken salad somewhere. Or, when I had to grab lunch in Dublin city centre recently, I went to a Mexican restaurant and got a bowl of healthy food – brown rice, beans, pulled chicken and spinach with no sauce.

When I'm travelling to an evening event I'll often get dinner there and I'll have no idea what it's going to be. But whatever dinner has been laid on, I'll generally go for meat and veg or fish and veg. I'll skip the potatoes and add extra veg, and I'll also skip dessert. That's pretty much it until tomorrow.

Again, this is an ideal day when things are going well. I don't always succeed because sometimes life throws you a curve ball, and maybe you've no option but to eat at a service station or raid a vending machine. But this is the kind of eating I aspire to every day and that I try to make happen. I truly believe intention is an important aspect to all things related to diet. If you *intend* to eat healthily you'll find you'll eat healthily 70–80 per cent of the time. However, if you don't even set an intention, that's when you'll find yourself regularly eating any old crap with zero nutritional value and zero value for your sleep.

WHEN TO EAT

Timing is everything. Everyone contends with their own sleep nemesis. I have a few, but the biggest one for me is eating late at night. From my research, the advice I have found and what I do believe to be true is: don't eat for three hours before bedtime, and don't have that bedtime snack.

Recently, I had a horrible night's sleep. I had an event in Portugal and the flight got me in pretty late. But I still thought I had enough time; it was 9 p.m., when I'd planned to eat, and I was going to go to bed at midnight and get up at 8 a.m.

I was staying in the town of Lousã and I went out to find a restaurant. Eating options were limited because it was all little coffee shops and bars. But I found a restaurant and went in, only to be told they had no space. Now it's 9.30 p.m., and I have to walk back to the hotel, I'm really hungry and I have no food with me. I ordered room service, but the menu was all very traditional Portuguese and very meat-heavy – not the sort of food I'd usually eat at night. I got a veal burger and chips, which arrived to my room at 10.45. Maybe I just shouldn't have eaten but I was so hungry I did, and I had the worst night's sleep that I had in a year. Lesson learned.

To a degree, you have to be regimented about your food and when you eat. Everybody has their own food journey and for me, I know what my cut-off time is – three hours before I go to bed – and I absolutely cannot eat after that, because if I do I'm not going to get a restful night's sleep.

The formula I would like you to try is:
> Dinner – three hours before bed
> A warm uncaffeinated drink – 1–2 hours before bed
> Small glass of water, if required – just before bed.

I bet you're still wondering about Paddy, the successful businessman who came to me for help. I'm happy to report that Paddy's rash is gone, he is no longer smoking cigarettes and he's getting seven to eight hours of solid sleep every single night. Paddy is one of my great success stories, and here's the thing: you can be too.

4

THE GLOWING ORB OF RELAXATION

In this, the last chapter in the Physical section of the book, you're going to learn more about visualisation, and a Sleep Hack that can induce deep relaxation, no matter how stressed you feel.

A WORLD OF WORRY

Everyone has days when the weight of the world seems to rest on your shoulders. Stress and tension cling to you, making a good night's sleep seem an impossible goal. You're mentally wound up; you're physically wound up. We've all been there. But you know what? I've learned over the years how to physically relax my body, which then leads to a calming of the mind. I've shared this technique with hundreds of clients and almost every one of them has achieved a similar outcome.

Every single thought we have sets off a series of physiological responses in the body and we are carrying more tension in our bodies now than at any other time in history. This is mainly as a result of the high levels of the fight or flight stress hormone cortisol, flooding our biochemistry every day. We are constantly stressed out – stressed about work, our kids, war, climate change, what to eat, what not to eat – and rushing from meeting to meeting. One 'expert' telling you to be a vegan, the next expert telling you to be a carnivore. Information, misinformation, conspiracy theories, negative news – it's all seeping in for hours and hours every single day!

We're worried about the cost of living. We're worried about the potential of another recession. We're worried the next storm might damage our house. Parents are worried that their kids might be being bullied online. We're unknowingly stressed on a subconscious level from the amount of content we're absorbing online all the time. These stress points and worries can have a devastating impact on our overall health and physiology. If you find yourself immersed in the pages of this book, it's evident that concerns about the insufficient amount or compromised quality of your sleep weigh heavily on your mind, hindering your ability to experience a restful night's sleep. It's all a bit of a vicious circle because poor sleep will raise your stress levels. One study from the University of California, Berkeley found that missing just one night's sleep increases emotional stress by 30 per cent.[17] That's *huge*! As a brain hacker, I know what you're thinking: 'That's not me'; or 'I'm very productive on low amounts of sleep.' Take a step back for a moment and think about when you were last in a bad mood. Or had an argument. Or skipped your exercise. If you are honest with yourself those moments are most likely triggered by lack of quality sleep. This means you're putting your mental health in jeopardy by missing just one night's sleep. That may seem like scaremongering, but it's really not. I'm laying down the facts as I have them and both you and I need a reality check. We need to prioritise our sleep. Not only that – we need to make it our number one priority. As you continue to read through these chapters you'll discover why it should become the most important habit in your life. There's a biological reason why your stress levels increase after even one night of insufficient sleep. Studies have shown that sleep deprivation leads to a 37–45 per cent increase in cortisol levels.[18] High cortisol levels are necessary when you're in a dangerous situation and you need your body to go into alarm mode, but clearly this is the last thing you need when you want to go to sleep.

MIND OVER BODY

In order to get a good night's rest, we must learn how to release the tension in our physical bodies and also reduce our stress hormones. The great news is that everyone has the ability to use their mind to induce relaxation in the body and in turn reduce not only their cortisol levels but also adrenaline and norepinephrine. Adrenaline and norepinephrine increase heart rate and blood pressure as part of the body's response to stress. By reducing these stress hormones, the body can return to a more normal, restful state, allowing the heart rate and blood pressure to decrease, which is essential for initiating and maintaining sleep.

A few years ago I was in Los Angeles. The morning after a late-night appearance on *The Jimmy Kimmel Show*, having had very little sleep, I was driving out of a parking spot and out of nowhere spotted a car speeding down the wrong side of the road and about to smash into me. I braked and somehow the other car managed to narrowly avoid me. But something went off in my brain and out of character my middle finger went up and I flipped off the driver of the other car. As my finger was in mid-air I noticed what he looked like. Anger turned to fear as I noticed he had a shaved head and his whole head and face were covered in gangland tattoos. The message from my brain to my hand wasn't fast enough to get my hand down. As I turned right to go to the gym I heard his brakes screech. I knew what was about to happen. My heart raced. My face tingled. He reversed his car at speed as I tried to get away. All of a sudden I realised I was in a high-speed car chase with what I was assuming was a gangland criminal. I turned right onto Pico Boulevard and got stuck at a red light where it intersects La Cienega. I was stuck with nowhere to go. He pulled up beside me in his red Ford Mustang and rolled down his window. As he screamed, 'Why you cuss me off like that, you little bitch? I'll pop you right now, motherfucker', he waved his handgun through the window. I froze, slowly raised my hands and mouthed 'Please don't shoot.' He swung his car around and sped off. When the light went green I proceeded, shaking like a leaf caught in a windstorm. I pulled over as soon as I could. As the shakes subsided I began to laugh. I laughed and laughed and laughed like a crazy person. Happy to be alive. Happy to have simply survived.

When we have a sad thought we cry, when we think of something funny we laugh, when we have a scary thought we get a reddening of the skin. Sometimes these physiological changes are so tiny they can be difficult to spot, but nonetheless I think we can all agree that our mind can have a profound impact on our physiology.

In our intricate biological system, the chemical responses to laughter and fear share some remarkable similarities. Both emotions trigger the release of neurotransmitters, which act as messengers in our body. Moments of humour or joy stimulate the release of neurotransmitters such as dopamine and endorphins. These chemicals contribute to a feeling of happiness and pleasure.

On the flip side, when we experience fear or a sudden fright, our body initiates the release of stress hormones, including adrenaline and cortisol. These hormones prepare the body for a 'fight or flight' response by increasing heart rate, sharpening our senses, and redirecting energy to essential functions.

Now here's where it gets interesting. While the specific neurotransmitters and hormones associated with laughter and fear are different, the pathways they travel are closely interconnected. The brain doesn't have separate pipelines for these emotions; instead, it navigates through a shared network. This can lead to intriguing moments where a surprising or unexpected event, like a twist in a comedy or a jump scare in a horror movie, or in my case a gun being drawn on me, elicits a mixed response.

In essence, our body's chemical responses to laughter and fear are like two sides of the same coin, closely related yet distinctly expressed, showcasing the fascinating complexity of our emotional and physiological experiences.

TRY THIS: MEMORY MAGNIFICATION

› Close your eyes and think of a funny memory. The funniest memory you can think of.
› As you visualise this memory, gently touch your tongue to the roof of your mouth.
› Magnify the memory and add in as many details as you can remember.

> Hold on to this memory for 60 seconds and then open your eyes and relax your tongue.
> Repeat daily or as often as you wish. Here's the fun part – after doing this several times the memory will be associated with your tongue pressing against the roof of your mouth. Any time you want to change your mental state and feel happy before bedtime, simply press your tongue to the roof of your mouth to naturally decrease your stress hormones and increase your feel-good hormones.

DRAWING A MENTAL PICTURE

A study carried out at Ohio University showed how powerful mental imagery can be in commanding our physical bodies to respond to our thoughts.[19]

A total of 29 people took part in the experiment. All 29 people had their wrists on their non-dominant forearm/wrist immobilised for four weeks using a lightweight polyethylene cast. Of the 29 people, 14 were instructed to use mental imagery (visualisation) five days a week over the four-week period, with the other 15 people acting as a control group.

During the days the test group used their visualisation techniques, they were asked to imagine contracting their wrist 52 times. Every time they were asked to imagine the contraction for five seconds, followed by a five-second rest. They imagined they were contracting maximally against a wrist grip and that they were pushing really hard against it. At the end of the four weeks the researchers were stunned to discover that the people who had imagined their wrists getting stronger had wrists twice as strong as the control group!

This is truly mind-blowing. If we can actually increase our strength using the power of the mind alone, imagine how much we can relax the physical body in preparation for sleep.

It therefore makes complete sense that we can also use our mind to relax our muscles, nerves and tendons to prepare for a night of tranquil sleep.

SO HOW ARE YOU FEELING?

Start now by asking yourself how you physically feel when you hit the pillow. Do you feel exhausted? Fatigued? Tense? Achy?

According to Chronic Pain Ireland, the national charity providing information and support services to people living with chronic pain, up to 1 in 3 adults in Ireland wake up most days with chronic pain, which is pain that persists for more than three months. The Irish Pain Society estimates that 42 per cent of people living in Ireland with chronic pain think others doubt the existence of their pain, even though 21 per cent said their pain was so intense they wanted to die. As well as having a devastating impact on individuals, chronic pain also has a societal cost in terms of healthcare and lost productivity: the Irish Pain Society estimates that chronic pain costs the Irish economy around €4.7 billion per year.

It's difficult to diagnose, it's highly variable and it's difficult to treat. One of the largest longitudinal studies of chronic pain in Ireland is the PRIME study (Prevalence, Impact and Cost of Chronic Non-Cancer Pain in Ireland in Adults), which was published in 2011. Conducted by the Centre for Pain Research at NUI Galway, which incidentally is where I went to college, the study surveyed

3,136 people in Ireland, and 35 per cent of those surveyed reported pain that met the International Association of the Study of Pain's definition of chronic pain. It also found that the average duration of pain reported was 7.6 years, but it ranged from 3 months to 50 years. Those who have chronic pain were five times more likely to be clinically depressed, and 12 per cent were unable to work full-time.

Why am I mentioning all this? First, because so many people are affected by chronic pain, and even if that pain isn't diagnosed as chronic, a lot of people will have aches and sprains and pulled muscles, or some discomfort. Whatever your level of pain or discomfort, even if it's almost unnoticeable, you can use what I call the Glowing Orb of Relaxation, which we'll come to in a moment, to help alleviate that pain; and that will by default lead to a deeper night's sleep. It's a win–win situation. The other reason I mention it is that I have an admission.

Technically, I should be one of those people diagnosed with chronic pain.

The car crash that I mentioned earlier in this book, the accident that set me on this path of improving my sleep, left me with injuries that continue to hurt to this day; I still also have residual pain in my ankle and left leg due to the accident. I'm in quite a lot of pain on a daily basis. I manage that pain without medication, utilising the power of my mind, and I try to 'physiotherapy' my way out of everything, but that's not always possible. I've got impingements under both shoulders, which are basically pinched tendons and trapped fluid in the shoulder joints. Every time I do a certain action, they click and give me a jolt of pain. I also have what's called fisherman's elbow. This is the degeneration of the tendon that's attached to the bony part of the elbow. It's incredibly painful and a lot of rod and line anglers get it. Needless to say, I'm not fishing very often at the moment. Then there's the tear and the cyst in my right wrist from a fall in Wexford Opera House (walking up the stairs while staring at my phone!). Out of nowhere I've just been diagnosed with a hernia in my groin to add to my ongoing list of injuries, and this will have to be operated on. I also thought I might have had a degenerative disc in my lower back, as it completely seizes up on occasion. Thankfully, it's not a disc issue but a muscular spasm. Still, when it happens, I have to see if I can make it to a bed or lie down somewhere, and I'll be like that for two days.

My body has also been affected by all the crazy stunts that I've done over the years. As part of the first series of *The Keith Barry Experience* in 2018, I did an escape where I was hanging upside down from a crane outside the RTÉ buildings, about 150 feet in the air. I was restrained in a straitjacket, with my head wrapped in clingfilm so I couldn't see or breathe and I was thrashing around violently while attempting to escape. Getting out of a straitjacket is really difficult. There's a myth that you have to dislocate your shoulder to do it. That's not actually true. But you do have to contort your body into all kinds of strange positions. On that day I had a major problem getting out of the straitjacket and I twisted myself badly somehow. I didn't know at the time, but a couple of weeks later I discovered that I had detached the cartilage from my left ribcage. Because I'd waited so long to go to a doctor about it (suffering from the stupid hard man syndrome I learned as a child in school in Waterford), the cartilage had knitted itself back onto the bone again in a very strange position. If I had sought medical help in time, they would have been able to operate, but doctors aren't able to do anything about it now. As a result, I always have pain in my ribcage.

So I always have some level of pain, full stop. It impacts my life in different ways – my ribcage even hurts when I wipe myself after going to the toilet! But, as I mentioned, I don't take painkillers and I rely on the power of my mind to deal with the pain.

One of my go-to tools to relax my body and to also reduce the effect of pain on my body is the Glowing Orb of Relaxation. I first devised this around 15 years ago. It's a serene sanctuary that you carry within yourself and a place of tranquillity that's always there, just waiting for you to unlock it. It's highly effective not only to reduce pain but also to relax the body in preparation for sleep.

TRY THIS: NIGHT-TIME TENSION-RELIEF DANCE

> Around 30 minutes before bedtime put on your favourite relaxation music and have a five-minute spontaneous dance session.
> Allow your body to move freely with no thought – just move in a relaxed and flowing motion with the music.
> Slow your body down for the final minute so you are barely moving at all. Still in flow with the music, just really, really slow.

Doing this can be a fun and liberating method for releasing tension and inducing relaxation in the body.

MEET LULU

Before I explain the Glowing Orb of Relaxation technique, allow me to introduce you to Lulu. I met Lulu through one of my shows for a TV network in the US. I'd designed an experiment based solely around sleep for the show and I wanted to test it out. What I needed was someone who had deep, long-standing issues with sleep, and so I contacted a renowned sleep centre in Los Angeles. Speaking to sleep experts there, I asked them if they could help me find somebody who had had treatment at the centre, but who still struggled with sleep, despite the myriad of techniques at the disposal of the sleep centre. They introduced me to Lulu. She was, at that time, in her late 50s and she was a complete and utter chronic insomniac, to the extent that she kept falling asleep behind the wheel of her car. In fact, she'd already had three car accidents because of her insomnia. The lack of sleep was detrimental to her mental health, as well as her physical health. There was a good chance that if her sleep problems weren't solved, she was going to die or even kill somebody else. Lulu had tried medication, but for whatever reason this hadn't helped her insomnia.

She came along to the sleep centre. I wanted to do this experiment under test conditions, in front of scientists as well as a camera crew. Because it was an entertainment show, there was also a mentalism demonstration aspect to it too.

The first thing I did was give her a book – it just happened to be a nature book – and I asked her to read it on camera. She read it relatively fast, over the course of about 90 minutes. Then she put the book under her pillow on her bed in the sleep centre. Next, I guided her through the Glowing Orb of Relaxation technique. Before I got to the end of the technique, which was just going to be part of the physical relaxation process before I began to use deep, hypnotic language, Lulu fell asleep. We could see her brainwave patterns because she was hooked up to an EEG machine, which measures electrical activity in the brain.

Typically, when Lulu fell asleep, she would wake up within the hour. Six hours later, the camera crew was still there, and I was eagerly waiting for her to wake up. Everybody was asking the one question I couldn't answer – how long is this lady going to sleep for? The sleep centre staff said the production team were going to have to leave, as they were closing for the night, although Lulu could stay there sleeping.

We decided to wake Lulu, and I very gently brought her out of her deep sleep. She felt wonderful. She had dreamt vividly that she was in a forest for the whole time, walking around barefoot on lush green grass.

This all happened because of the power of the Glowing Orb of Relaxation.

Let's dive deep into this concept. I've been on stages, in people's minds, and now I want to take you on a journey inside yourself.

The first thing to note is that relaxation is a skill and it's one you can master – it's like getting to the top of your game at a sport or learning a new language. It just needs dedication, patience and the right mindset. We often get so caught up in our daily routines and responsibilities that we neglect our own wellbeing. But taking care of yourself is not a luxury; it's a necessity.

One of the keys to unlocking the Glowing Orb of Relaxation technique is mindfulness. It's about being completely present in the moment and focusing entirely on what's happening right here, right now. Mindfulness is like a superpower that allows you to fully embrace the present moment.

Remember that relaxation and freedom from pain isn't a destination; it's a continuous journey. It's about recognising that regardless of what's going on in your life, or how stressful things might be, you possess an inner sanctuary of relaxation, and you have the Glowing Orb of Relaxation at your disposal.

When I'm on stage, there's a similar feeling. It's that electrifying moment just before a grand illusion unfolds. The audience is in suspense, and I can feel their energy. But there's a unique kind of relaxation in that moment. I've practised, I've prepared, and I'm entirely present. That's when magic happens.

Now it's your turn to create your magic.

THE POWER OF VISUALISATION

One of the greatest tools I've discovered along my journey is the power of visualisation. It's like a mental rehearsal for relaxation. You can achieve remarkable results by vividly picturing your desired outcomes. That's across the board, whether it's acing a job interview, conquering a fear or achieving deep, restorative sleep. Visualisation is your secret weapon.

The colour purple is integral to this technique. Why? I discovered early on in my career that when I have someone on stage and I'm trying to get them into a deep stage of relaxation and slow down their brainwaves, exposure to the colour purple works every time. Colour psychology says purple is often associated with qualities like peace, tranquillity and spirituality, which is why it's such a relaxing hue.

When you first try this technique, you might be thinking, 'How do I know if I'm doing it right?' The truth is, there's no one 'right' way to visualise. It's a deeply personal experience, and the key is to let go of expectations. Your mind knows the way; you just need to trust it.

TRY THIS: GIVE YOURSELF A HUG In preparation for an amazing night's sleep, I want you to do something first before we get into the details of the Glowing Orb of Relaxation.

I want you to give yourself a glowing hug.

What that means is you close your eyes and you remember a time when somebody hugged you and you felt really good about that. It could be a parent, a teacher, a friend, a sister, a brother, a niece or nephew, your child or your partner. It can be anybody you want – just remember a moment where you felt safe and secure in somebody's arms. This can go all the way back to childhood, or it can be as recent as yesterday, but it is a moment when you felt loved. Then place your hand on your heart.

Now imagine that moment in the colour purple. And as you imagine that moment on the screen in your head in the colour purple, just allow yourself to bask in the power of that moment for approximately 60 seconds. Hold on to that picture in your mind; feel the feelings of that hug for an entire minute. Live that memory in your mind.

There's solid science as to why I want you to do this first. Hugs release the chemical oxytocin, sometimes called the 'cuddle hormone'. Oxytocin makes us feel less stressed and makes us feel good about ourselves; it's the chemical of bonding, affection and attachment. Essentially, we associate oxytocin with happiness, and it reduces stress hormones and lowers our blood pressure. There are other health benefits too. In one study of over 400 people, scientists looked at the effect hugging had as a stress buffer in susceptibility to colds.[20] Participants were exposed to a common cold virus and monitored for signs of illness. The study found that those who felt socially supported and were hugged more experienced fewer signs of illness. Hugs can also help with pain. In another study of people with fibromyalgia syndrome, a chronic disorder that causes pain and tenderness in the body, as well as fatigue and difficulty sleeping, scientists discovered that therapeutic touch resulted in an increase of quality of life and reduced pain for participants – and hugging is a form of therapeutic touch.

One of the most vocal proponents of hugs is American academic Professor Paul Zak. He's a regular TED speaker and he helped start several interdisciplinary fields including neuromarketing and neuro-economics. He has been nicknamed Dr Love by the media, and he is an oxytocin expert. He calls oxytocin the 'moral molecule' because when someone is nice to you, your oxytocin levels go up, and this causes you to be nicer. This has been shown in subjects who were given an artificial oxytocin via an inhaler, and who subsequently behaved in a nicer fashion. Oxytocin connects us to other people, he says, and makes us feel what other people feel.

In his book *The Moral Molecule: The Source of Love and Prosperity*, he writes:

> *Let Dr Love offer you a prescription: eight hugs a day. We've shown that if you give eight hugs a day you'll be happier, and the world will be a better place because you'll be causing others' brains to release oxytocin. They, in turn, will connect better to others, treat them more generously, causing oxytocin release ... yes, the virtuous cycle begins with a hug.*

Real-life, physical self-hugs also stimulate oxytocin production, so a self-hug definitely counts, as does hugging a pet. And of course, visualising a hug where all was right in your world and you felt calm and secure works just as well, as the power of your mind and that memory is enough to activate the release of oxytocin. When released, oxytocin can have a calming effect on the nervous system, reducing stress and anxiety levels. This physiological response can be particularly beneficial for people struggling with sleep difficulties. Incorporating self-hugging into a pre-sleep routine will contribute to a more relaxed state of mind and body. This heightened sense of calmness can pave the way for a smoother transition into sleep, fostering a good night's rest. Embracing the therapeutic potential of self-hugging may offer a simple yet effective way to harness the natural mechanisms in the body to improve sleep quality.

Now that you've given yourself a glowing hug (and I recommend you do it nightly), you are ready to move on to the Glowing Orb of Relaxation technique.

SLEEP HACK 6
THE GLOWING ORB OF RELAXATION

An audio recording where I guide you through this visualisation can be accessed on my website www.keithbarry.com/sleephacks with the password SLEEPHACKS24.

> - Lie down and close your eyes.
> - Take three long, relaxing deep breaths, in and out.
> - Imagine for a moment you're lying on a beach late at night, listening to the waves crash on the shore and looking up towards the beautiful sky, enjoying gazing at the stars and

the empty space between the stars. As you gaze at those stars you notice a purple light, about the size of a hot air balloon, hovering among them. The moment you begin to gaze at that light you notice your mind, body and soul start to relax completely and fully. You are inquisitive about this purple light as it gently moves closer to you.

› After just a few moments the light moves so close that you can see it in full detail and you just stare and observe it for just a few moments. As you look at that purple light, you notice how soft and tranquil it seems and how comfortable it might be for you to just walk right inside that purple orb.

› The moment you enter that purple glow, you immediately find yourself relaxing a thousand times more. Now you notice the only other object in that glowing purple orb is an inviting and sumptuous bed. You just want to gently slip into that bed. As you do so – and it feels amazing – you notice the soothing purple light surrounding you. As you sink down into the bed, you observe that you are relaxing even more. Bathed in purple light, your legs begin to get heavier, your arms get heavier and you just melt into the bed.

› And now you notice how you can begin to draw that purple light into your body. Begin with your lower limbs, and visualise that purple light entering through your toes and into your feet. As you notice that purple light moving into your feet, it guides you deeper and deeper into a wonderful state of pure relaxation. And now allow that purple light to enter into your ankles and your shins. Make every effort to actually allow your ankles and shins to completely relax. But also now imagine the purple light entering into those parts of your body that have aches and pains. And the moment you visualise the purple light entering into the parts of your body that have those aches and pains, just allow those aches and pains to dissipate and notice immediately how they actually disappear.

- Continue moving that blissful purple light up through your body, making an effort to only focus on that particular part of the body where the light is and allowing that part of your body to soften, loosen and relax. Bring that purple light up through your stomach, into your chest, and as the light enters different parts of your body, allow that part of your body to become more relaxed, soft and at ease.

- Continue to do this for every part of your body. Once it has been absorbed into your external body, now imagine that purple light as your breath. As you inhale that purple light, visualise that purple light entering your lungs and allow your lungs to relax. Now it spreads through your lungs into your spleen, your heart, your liver, your kidneys, allowing all of those to settle and work in unison. Yesterday is gone, tomorrow is a new day. In this moment, right here, right now, nothing matters except pure, wonderful relaxation, allowing your autonomic nervous system to settle down as that purple light travels through your bloodstream into every cell in your body. Just allow every part of your physiological body to settle down and relax even more.

- Once you've allowed that purple light from that glowing sphere to enter into every muscle, nerve, fibre and cell in your body, repeat these affirmations in your mind silently to yourself and keep repeating these positive messages:

> *I am safe and relaxed*
> *My body is ready to rest and heal*
> *I am safe and relaxed*
> *My body is ready to rest and heal.*
> Relax, take a deep breath, and let that Glowing Orb of Relaxation envelop you. You've got this.

I have so many examples over the years of how the Glowing Orb of Relaxation has helped people to physically relax, often as a precursor to one of my wild hypnotic demonstrations. In one of my shows in the US, it worked a treat in paving the way for one of my subjects to believe he was a sleeper agent – a spy who was undercover and who could be activated to do something once he saw a particular visual or audio cue. I advertised for people to come on a show, which was being billed as a sleep show, where I would be doing sleep experiments. This particular applicant was a student in his mid twenties, and I arranged to meet him at a warehouse. Although the surroundings might have seemed strange, he'd been warned to expect the unexpected. After using the Glowing Orb of Relaxation to relax his physical body I then induced him into a deep trance and used hypnotic language to plant the seed that he was a sleeper agent. When I finally brought him out of the trance, he thought he'd dreamed that he had visited a coffee shop and planted a poisonous pill in the drink of a particular man – a defecting government agent – before picking up a briefcase containing classified information, and leaving the coffee shop. It wasn't until he saw the video evidence and the briefcase beside his bed in the warehouse that he realised he had actually done all this (the coffee shop was full of actors who were aware of the experiment). He was a little shocked – to say the least – that he could actually be turned into a sleeper agent via hypnotic language, and be brought out of that mental state and think it was a dream. My point is that the Glowing Orb of Relaxation had relaxed him into a very deep state of relaxation, a state that he couldn't ordinarily achieve, as he was someone who struggled with relaxing. And that then, through hypnosis, I placed the idea that he was a sleeper agent and then he acted on that idea.

Another of my favourite examples of the potency of the glowing orb of relaxation is when I went to South Africa ten years ago to film what turned out to be an award-winning ad for an insurance company. José, my assistant of over twenty years, and I headed to Johannesburg. One of our security personnel there was a man called Xander, and we got on particularly well with him. I had to do castings to find people who would be hypnotisable for the ad and I hypnotised hundreds and hundreds of people around Johannesburg. Xander was watching this the whole time and he was observing me putting people to sleep every single day.

It was only on the final day when we were leaving that Xander piped up and said he had a favour to ask. He said: 'I have really bad insomnia. What I've seen you do here the last five days, it just looks like a miracle, putting all these different people to sleep. Can you help me? Can you hypnotise me to sleep?' Of course I said yes. We were travelling back to the airport at this point – Xander wasn't driving, by the way; he and José were in the back of the car together – and the first thing I did with him was the Glowing Orb of Relaxation. As I was using the Glowing Orb on Xander, José fell asleep, then Xander fell asleep and they were snoring horrendously out of sync. I couldn't wait to get out of the car!

Crafted to induce physical relaxation as a prelude to sleep, the Glowing Orb technique also has the potential to seamlessly usher you into a profound state of slumber. Beyond its intended purpose of soothing the body, the very engagement with this method might prove sufficient to lull you into a restful and rejuvenating sleep experience.

Interestingly, José hadn't used this technique before; now he is still using the Glowing Orb to get him into a deep state of relaxation before going to sleep. We also got an email from Xander a month later saying that he'd had the most beautiful nights of sleep since.

And what about Lulu? You're probably wondering how she got on.

Six months after she took part in the sleep experiment I got the loveliest Facebook message from her. She said that she'd been sleeping eight hours every single night ever since and she was very grateful. Not only that, to loop back to what I mentioned in the first chapter, Lulu realised that there was a lot more to life for her. In other words, she had found her subconscious 'why'. She was more productive, she was happier, she was more content. Her mental wellbeing had improved, her physical health was significantly better, and she was no longer scared of getting behind the wheel. Her whole life had changed since that one day. That was a really poignant moment for me.

You may also be wondering what the mentalism demonstration I performed on Lulu was. After she woke up and described her dream in detail I instructed her to look inside the pillow she had been sleeping on for hours. Inside the pillow was a sketch which described the exact dream sequence she had just had. How did I do it? Using hypnotic language I manipulated her dreams so she actually had a specific dream that I had put inside her mind. I will describe in detail later how you can also manipulate your own dreams to help you solve problems and increase your creativity.

Remember: This is only one of the relaxation techniques for you to use. If you don't like it for some reason, try the others. If you do like it, and it's working for you, you can stick with it, or you can mix up the techniques. It's whatever feels comfortable for you and whatever works for you.

GLOWING ORB OF RELAXATION: FOUR STEPS TO REMEMBER

1. Give yourself a glowing hug.
2. Visualise a purple orb floating from the night sky and drifting towards you. As it gets closer and closer you immediately begin to relax.
3. Imagine yourself slipping into a sumptuous bed inside the orb, safe in the relaxing glow of the glowing purple orb.
4. Visualise the glowing purple light entering into every muscle, nerve and fibre, beginning at your feet and moving up your body. Then, when you are completely immersed in the purple light, repeat your positive affirmations.

Just as a little reminder, you've now finished the Physical section of the book. Before moving on to the Psychological section, remember that you are going to select one of the Physical Sleep Hacks, numbered 1–6) and commit to it daily.

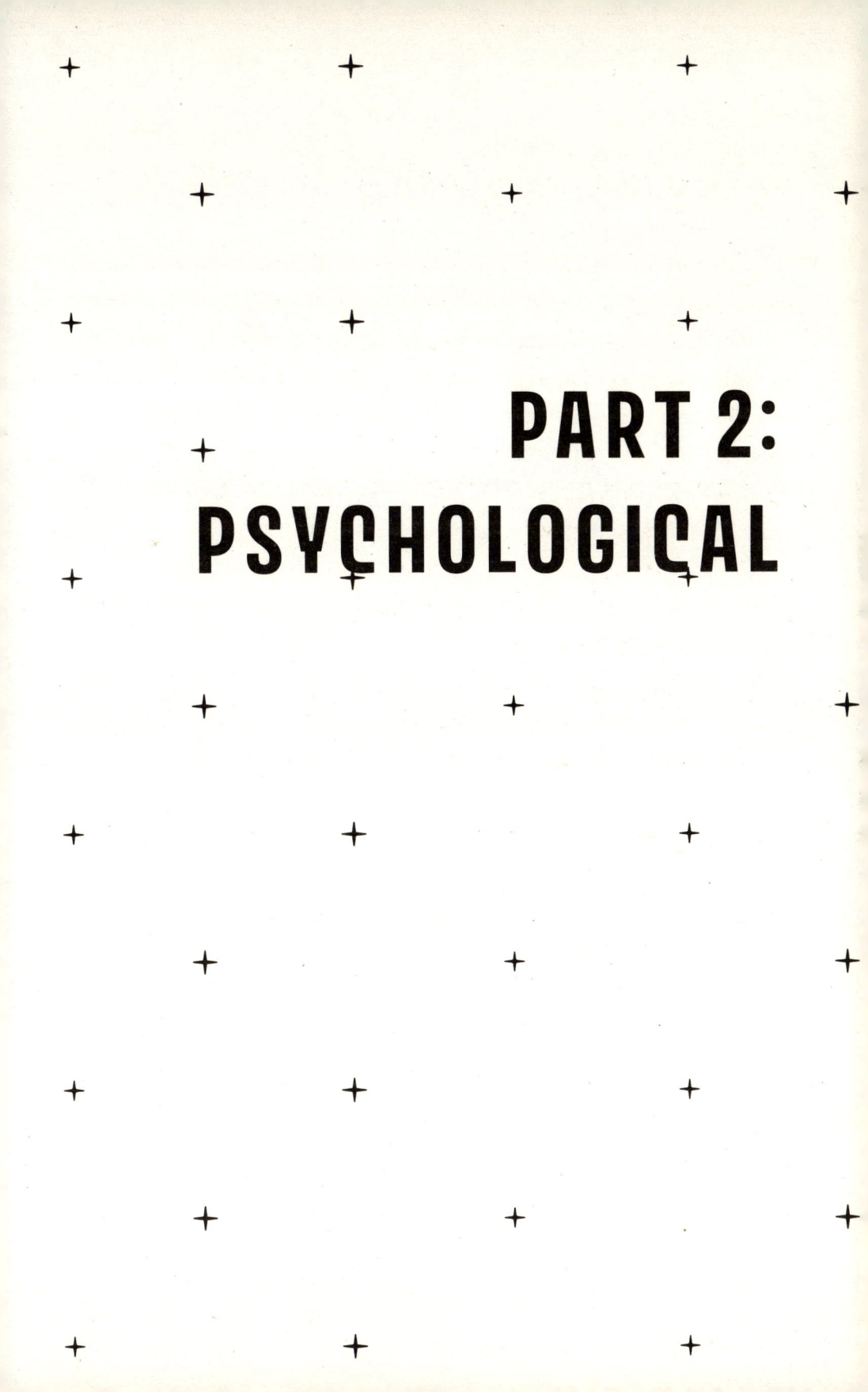

PART 2: PSYCHOLOGICAL

5

LOOK INTO MY EYES

In the previous chapters, I've showed you ways to relax your physical body, techniques that can calm and soothe your physiology, and how to prep your body for sleep. But this is only one segment of creating your own unique sleep system.

The next step is to settle your conscious mind, to help your mind relax so that your body can do what it is supposed to do at nighttime. Over the next three chapters, you'll read nine different Sleep Hacks that will help calm your mind and help you get an excellent night's sleep – and you only have to choose one of them.

SETTLING YOUR CONSCIOUS MIND

What is the conscious mind? It's a question that has frustrated scientists and, in truth, it's something that for a long time concerned philosophers more than scientists. At a very basic level, your conscious mind is everything you're aware of and that you're thinking about. But it's quite hard to define and even harder to study objectively and to figure out what parts of the brain are neurologically involved in 'awareness'. Without digging too deeply into all of these, for the purposes of your sleep, the conscious mind needs to be quietened and settled in order for you to sleep. That means not thinking about your next payday or the parent–teacher meeting you have to attend tomorrow. The active brain needs to be lulled into a calm and peaceful state, and over the next few chapters I'm going to share strategies for how you can do this.

Harnessing the power of hypnotism has played an important part in my career. Hypnotism fascinates most people, as it appears almost magical when a person instantly falls into a deep hypnotic sleep with the mere use of words. Some of the techniques in this book use the power of self-hypnosis to help guide you into a deep night's rest. Hence, it's important you understand the background of hypnosis to fully appreciate the power it can have and also to help alleviate any concerns or scepticism you may have regarding its use as a sleep aid. The practice, as we now know it, started to emerge in the late nineteenth century. But its history is far older than that. More than four thousand years ago there were sleep temples dedicated to the Egyptian priest Imhotep. These were healing sanctuaries where people would go to be cured of both physical and mental ailments. Patients were put into a hypnotic state and influenced by suggestions before falling asleep, and their treatment was often based on a priest's interpretation of their dreams.

The ancient Greeks also knew how important sleep is for wellbeing. They too had sleep temples, which were dedicated to Asclepius, the god of medicine. These were places of healing, built in the fifth and fourth centuries BCE, where priests used chants to put patients into a trance-like state known as 'incubation' (from the Latin *in* (on) and *cubare* (to lie)). People would travel for hundreds of miles to partake in these sleep rituals and sleep in a sacred space, to receive a divinely inspired cure or the answer to a conundrum.

Over three hundred sleep temples or asclepieia have been found throughout ancient Greece. At one of them, the Asclepieion of Epidaurus, you can see marble tablets dating from 350 BCE that capture the names of 70 patients, their histories, medical problems and cures undertaken while the patient was in a dream-like state of induced sleep.

It's clear that people in ancient times recognised the powerful healing properties of sleep, and how hypnosis can be a route to that.

Fast forward to more relatively recent times, and there's a long list of people who developed the practice to its more recognisable form today. These include the German doctor Franz Mesmer, who developed the concept of mesmerism. Mesmer believed that we all vibrate at certain frequencies and this energy, or 'animal magnetism', could be affected by passing magnets or even hands over a person's body to help realign their magnetic frequencies. There was a lot of controversy surrounding Mesmer and the validity of his methods, but there is no doubt that he contributed to the development of the field of 'mind over matter' and hypnosis. Scottish ophthalmologist James Braid introduced the term 'hypnotism' (from the Greek word for sleep, *hypnos*) in his book *Neurypnology; or, the Rationale of Nervous Sleep, Considered in Relation with Animal Magnetism* in 1843. He used the word 'hypnotism' to describe the state of focused attention and heightened suggestibility which someone could attain by staring at an object such as a pendulum or Braid's fingers as he waved them in front of their face. His vision was that hypnosis could be used to cure 'nervous' diseases and help patients in surgery with pain and anxiety.

Several scientific studies have found that hypnosis can help with sleep, with one from 2018 concluding that hypnosis for sleep problems is a promising treatment that warrants more investigation.[21] Another study found that hypnosis can extend slow-wave sleep, the type of sleep that is restorative.[22]

Even if you've never personally experienced hypnotism, you may be familiar with some of the methods hypnotists use to bring people into a deep state of relaxation. There's the classic 'look into my eyes' technique, popularised by stage hypnotists all over the world. The image of a swinging pocket watch has been synonymous with hypnotism, a technique known as 'eye fixation'. As you focus your gaze on the pendulum's graceful swing, you become deeply focused, your concentration intensifies, and gradually your eyes grow heavy with fatigue.

The eye fixation induction technique was originally developed by James Braid. It works on the principle of fixing your gaze on a specific point, while suggestions are given that your eyes are tired and you want to close them. The technique is threefold. First, doing this will physically make your eyes tired, as the eye muscles work constantly to maintain their position. Then, as you are focusing on a chosen point, your brain is engaged and becomes entranced, and this is quite physically soothing. Finally, as the hypnotist gives suggestions for relaxation, since the conscious mind is distracted, the suggestions are more readily accepted by the subconscious mind. When combined, these work collectively to relax the mind and body, making the subject more receptive to sleep.

I have hypnotised tens of thousands of people, but the traditional pocket watch is not part of my repertoire when I want to get someone to concentrate and focus. I have developed many different techniques to get people to focus on my commands and subsequently enter into deep trance. When it's part of one of my stage shows, I may ask the person to stare at a purple light on the stage (you can probably see how purple is a theme in my work). If it's in a one-to-one environment, I might ask them to look at my finger as a focal point, or maybe stare at the tip of a pen. This or any focal point serves as an entryway into the realm of deep relaxation and heightened suggestibility.

My own journey with hypnotism began when I was 14, and my sister Michele was my first subject. I'd picked up a book called *Practical Hypnotism* by Ed Wolff – it was first published in 1936, but you can still buy it today. On the front cover of that book there was a spiral pattern that I carefully cut out, as the book instructed. Placing it on a pin, I directed my sister to fixate her gaze on the spinning spiral as I gently rotated it with my finger. As she gazed at the hypnotic spiral, I calmly instructed her not to take her eyes away from it, that her eyelids were growing heavier with each passing second, and finally, in a soft whisper, I said, 'Sleep deep.' Her eyes closed and her head dropped forward. I thought she was messing with me. Play-acting and having a laugh. I lifted her arm from her leg and let it go. It flopped back down to her leg like a rag doll. I tried the other arm. Same thing. I gently lifted an eyelid and looked directly into her eye – no response. I then tried the ultimate test – I tickled her. Nothing. She was in a deep hypnotic trance. I gave her the suggestion that she would do something she would never ordinarily do – tidy up my room. When I brought her out of the trance she acted as if nothing had happened. I went out for a few hours with my friends. Lo and behold, when I came home my bedroom was spotless! Hoovered, polished and the bed made – I couldn't believe it! I told her I had hypnotised her but she was having none of it. It wasn't until the next day that she realised that she indeed had been hypnotised, and she reported that she had had the best night's sleep ever. After that, I was obsessed with hypnosis.

If you want to get a restful night's sleep, and you clearly do if you are reading this book, you can use the eye fixation technique to ensure your eyes are tired and your conscious mind is settled.

Sometimes clients tell me that they don't feel tired when they're going to bed, and maybe that's the case for you. You might feel too wired or stressed from the day, and you're feeling wide awake. What they need to do, and what you need to do, is to trick your mind and body that they are ready to sleep.

Now I want to show you how to utilise the technique of a hypnotist on yourself to prepare for a good night's sleep. This first technique is designed to gently tire your eyes out and soothe the mind.

SLEEP HACK 7
EYE FIXATION METHOD

FIND YOUR 'IMAGINED' SPOT

The first thing you need to do as you're lying in bed is to find an imagined spot in your room. Some people will have managed to get their bedroom completely dark, but most people can still see something in their room when they're in bed. If you can see a spot on the ceiling when you're in bed, focus on that spot. Maybe it's the glint of a lightbulb or even a mark on the ceiling – just pick anything you can find. If you can't see anything at all, simply imagine you can – this is why I call it an 'imagined' spot. Then I want you to gaze at this imagined spot. Gaze for as long as possible without blinking. Of course, when you really need to blink, do, but stare for as long as possible first. Next, imagine a thin purple line that goes from the end of your nose up to that imagined spot on the ceiling. This is an unbreakable purple thread that connects you to your imagined spot. It is an anchor that will keep your attention focused on this point. As you focus, you find your eyes beginning to become more and more relaxed as you look at the spot. You're not trying to blink but you're also not trying not to blink. You are just gazing at the spot, comfortably, blinking or not blinking as the case may be.

VISUALISE YOUR EYES BECOMING RELAXED

Visualise the muscles around your eyes becoming soft, loose and comfortable. Your eyelids will start to feel heavier and heavier, almost as if there are weights pulling them down. Any tension in your facial muscles that you might feel, any stress that you might feel in your forehead, just allow it to loosen and relax as you continuously gaze at that spot. You haven't been thinking about blinking, but now, every few seconds, you give yourself permission to blink gently. With every blink you take, you find that you begin to get more and more and more relaxed. Visualise each blink as a wave of soothing relaxation washing over you, not just your eyes but your entire body. Feel the relief that comes with every tranquil wave, allowing you to relax even more. Repeat the mantra silently over and over: *My eyelids are heavy. My eyelids are heavy. My eyelids are heavy.*

EXPERIENCE THE 'IMAGINED SPOT' BLENDING INTO THE BACKGROUND

As you continue to gaze at that spot on the ceiling, it will begin to dissipate, dissolve and disappear, inviting you into a deep state of wonderful, restful sleep. You might sense now that your eyes just want to close, as they begin to get heavier and heavier, so much so that it's difficult to keep them open. You just want to allow your eyes to shut down now and allow yourself to sink into a deep, inviting, wonderful sleep.

EYE FIXATION: FOUR STEPS TO REMEMBER

1. Find your imagined spot and visualise a thin purple line going from your nose to the spot.
2. Visualise your eyes relaxing, as if there are heavy weights on them.
3. Repeat the mantra silently to yourself *My eyelids are heavy* over and over.
4. Visualise the imagined spot blending into the background, as you prepare for a deep sleep.

There are other techniques I've developed over the years that follow a similar protocol as the eye fixation technique. The **zzz-infinity loop** technique is a brilliant way to distract the conscious mind and then subsequently programme the subconscious mind for sleep. It works because the mental exercise itself reduces conscious stimulation by focusing on contradictory thoughts and actions.

SLEEP HACK 8
THE ZZZ-INFINITY LOOP

> Begin by lying on your bed rather than in your bed so there is no resistance from your bedcovers. Imagine (with your eyes closed) a figure of eight infinity loop hovering in front of you. Picture this graceful symbol with its smooth curves about the size of a large pretzel. Use the index finger of your right hand to begin to trace the smooth curves of the infinity loop. Notice as it hovers in the air a trail of zzz's coming off the loop. As your finger traces the loop, allow your thoughts to quieten and just focus on maintaining contact with the imaginary figure of eight.

> Every time you complete a full loop with your finger, allow any other lingering thoughts to dissolve. Now stop moving your finger but keep it hovering in the centre of the loop. Begin to move your left foot in a circle, anti-clockwise. After completing five circles, start tracing your infinity loop with your finger once again and notice what happens to your foot. You'll notice that it's extremely difficult to do both simultaneously. Your focus here is to resist the mind–body conflict and attempt to accomplish the task at hand. The task is to complete 50 circles with your foot and 50 infinity loops with your finger. If you fail even once, you must begin again.

> Over the course of time you may indeed achieve this, so then begin with the opposing hand and leg. Once you can do both sides attempt to do both sides simultaneously.

Note: Whether or not you accomplish this task, it is designed to be done for no longer than five minutes. The concept here is to quieten the conscious mind by using a cognitive conflict as part of your pre-sleep shutdown process.

I was once in a fancy London establishment called Chiltern Firehouse with Woody Harrelson. We had been filming *Now You See Me 2* and went there for dinner one night. While in conversation with our waitress we told her that we were filming a magic movie where Woody was playing the part of a mentalist named Merritt. We explained that I was advising Woody on how to act like a mentalist/hypnotist and with an air of scepticism she said, 'I can't be hypnotised.' If I had a euro for every time someone said that to me, I'd have enough to buy a small tropical island and retire early! I asked her if she would give me permission to attempt to hypnotise her. When she agreed I immediately used my anti-gravity hands technique to induce relaxation in preparation for hypnosis. She was fascinated that her hands were floating up and away from her legs without her conscious awareness. The great news is you can use an adapted version of this technique as a sleep aid. Again, it acts as a subtle distraction for your conscious mind and also when you embed certain language inside your mind you will find yourself quickly getting dozy!

SLEEP HACK 9
ANTI-GRAVITY HANDS

> Settle into a comfortable position on your bed and allow your body to loosen and relax. Place your hands palms down on your legs. Turn your attention inwards and take a long, deep breath in and out, breathing in serenity and calmness, while exhaling any stress you've accumulated throughout the day.

- Bring your attention to your hands and imagine they are weightless, as if they are effortlessly floating in mid-air. Now with every breath you take, imagine your hands becoming lighter and lighter, completely and utterly weightless. Really make every effort to believe this is your current new reality. Begin to notice how your hands slowly and effortlessly rise from your legs of their own accord outside your conscious awareness. As your hands ascend, begin to associate this sensation with feelings of freedom and happiness. Freedom from any outside distractions and happiness in just being present in this moment.

- When your hands have floated up and into a comfortable position, notice how they stay suspended at that place of perfect buoyancy where gravity just seems to have lost its grip on them. Feel this moment and enjoy the delightful sensation released from the chains of the external world.

- Now let's try a contrasting experience. While they are still floating in space, turn your hands over and close them into fists. Imagine you are holding onto an empty bucket in each hand. In your mind begin to fill the buckets with water. Notice how the buckets begin to feel heavy and as a result your hands also begin to feel heavy. The more you breathe the heavier they become, and they begin to drift and sink slowly back down towards your legs.

- Really envision your hands transitioning from light to heavy, creating a balance of calmness and relaxation. When your hands eventually touch your legs again, allow that sensation of calmness and relaxation to spread into your legs and then from your legs into your entire body.

› Repeat this process five times, making every effort to allow your subconscious mind to take over from your conscious mind during the process.

You may be wondering what happened the waitress in the Chiltern Firehouse. I used the anti-gravity hands technique as we were sitting there chatting. Once her hands hit her legs, I immediately used a black ops induction technique to put her into a deep trance. This is a little-known underground hypnotic technique which I can't say too much about in this book. Suffice to say it's a technique developed by a secretive undercover governmental security force to literally take control of people's minds. The girl sat there, completely limp and motionless. Woody was freaked out. I then suggested to her that I was implanting a microchip in her arm so that I could take control of her arm at will. When I awakened her, she had no idea what had happened. Then I suggested to her that her hand was stuck to the table. Sure enough she could not lift it off the table. It was almost as if I had poured a tub of superglue over her hand and it had physically stuck to the table. Of course I then brought her out of trance and returned her back to normal. When I showed her footage of herself, she couldn't believe what she was seeing. After that, she was no longer a sceptic!

On Saturday 27 January 2024, I performed my largest indoor theatre show ever, with two thousand people packed into the Bord Gáis Energy Theatre in Dublin to witness *Mind Games*. I have a segment in the show where I need someone on stage who can easily fall into deep trance. So I do a series of susceptibility tests on the entire audience which essentially tells me who is most susceptible to hypnosis. As part of this sequence, I use a magnetic fingers test and then a magnetic hands test where people are invited to believe that their fingers and hands are magnets, and they are attracted to each other. To see two thousand people doing this is quite incredible. People are amazed that their fingers move together, seemingly of their own accord, underneath any level of cognitive awareness. Of course it doesn't work on everyone, but in my experience over 70 per cent of people have success with it.

SLEEP HACK 10
MAGNETIC FINGERS

> Interlock your hands together so your fingers are interlaced and hold your hands in front of your face. Squeeze your hands tightly together.
> Extend the index fingers of both hands so there is around an inch gap between them. Now take a long, relaxing deep breath in and out and imagine there are powerful magnets on the tips of your fingers. Notice how immediately the gap between your fingers begins to close and how magical it seems. The magnets in your mind are pulling your fingers closer and closer together until they eventually touch.
> When they touch, allow your hands to drop down and separate again.

There are two things happening here. First, due to your hand structure, your fingers physiologically want to move towards each other. More important, though, if you use your imagination properly and actually imagine the magnets, your subconscious mind will take over and move your fingers towards each other as if by magic.

SLEEP HACK 11
MAGNETIC HANDS TEST

The magnetic hands test is quite different, as we are relying solely on a psychological principle rather than physiological mixed with psychological. There is no physiological reason your hands will move towards each other, so if this works it is purely your subconscious mind taking over. This may not work the first time, and that's okay. What we want to achieve here is a state of focused attention and heightened awareness, so try it many times until you feel your subconscious taking over from your conscious mind.

- Sit in a quiet, comfortable place and decide to fully enter into this experience with an open, yet focused, state of mind. Take three long, deep breaths in and out and allow your mind to fully clear.
- Stretch your arms out in front of you with the palms of the hands facing each other.
- Imagine there are powerful magnets in the palms of your hands. Really make every effort to see these magnets in your mind's eye.
- Focus on the power of those magnets and you will notice your hands begin to move closer and closer together as if by magic. Do not consciously move your hands. Wait and allow your subconscious to accept the suggestion you are giving it. It may take some time, so be patient and wait until they begin to move. Generally this will take up to 60 seconds.
- When your hands eventually touch, allow them to separate and drop down gently, and inhale a deep breath of relaxation.

If you are one of the few people who this doesn't work for on the first try, be sure to try it multiple times until it does work.

After the two thousand people tried these tests, I progressed further by suggesting to the audience that their hands were locked together as if I had poured a large tub of superglue over them. Dozens of people in the audience accepted that suggestion and their hands indeed did glue together as if bonded by an imaginary force. When I gave the suggestion that their hands would unlock, I noticed giggles and laughter coming from the third level of the theatre. I cannot see that height due to the blinding theatre lights glaring from up there but figured out that one person's hands had not unlocked. I attempted to unlock them again from the stage, to no avail. I ran off the stage into the wings and sprinted as fast as I could up to the top level of the theatre. When I found the man whose hands would not separate it was insightful. His hands truly were stuck together as if an invisible force had fused and bonded them tightly. So there was only one thing for it. I gently touched his hands and said in a deep, paternal voice 'Sleep, deep, deep, sleep'. Instantly he dropped into a deep hypnotic trance. Fast asleep. Gone to the Land of Nod! It was magical to the audience – they freaked out as this man dropped instantly into a deep altered state of mind. We captured this moment on camera, so if you want to see it in action you'll find it on my Instagram page.

The reason I'm sharing this story with you is because you can use the magnetic hands principle to psychologically prepare you for sleep. Again, it acts as a focus point for your conscious mind and helps it settle in readiness for sleep.

This time we'll do it slightly differently:

- Lie down on your bed and take three long, deep breaths in and out. Allow your body to relax.
- Stretch your arms out in front of you, again with the palms of your hands facing each other.
- Take a moment to stare at your hands and imagine there are magnets attached to the palm of each hand.
- This time imagine the magnets are powerful relaxation magnets. Stare at your hands and focus on your breathing.
- Allow your hands to slowly move towards each other from the force of the magnets.
- When your hands eventually touch, use that as a mental bridge to fully relax your mind, body and soul in preparation for deep rest.
- Allow your hands to separate and rest down by your side.

Repeat as many times as necessary until you feel you are ready to sleep.

By the way, I do believe the man in the Bord Gáis would have stayed sound asleep for hours and missed the entire show if I hadn't woken him up. So just a few seconds later, I unstuck his hands and restored him back to normal in every single way, ready to enjoy the remainder of the show.

SLEEP HACK 12
SYNCHRONISED HARMONY FOR CONSCIOUS RELAXATION

This can be done seated or lying down, as long as you are comfortable and relaxed.

> Close your eyes and begin to notice the rhythm of your heart and the rhythm of your breath. Take time to really get in tune with your heartbeat and breath flow. Focus on slowing your heart rate and breathing simply through conscious intent.

> Begin to slowly tap your right foot gently on the surface beneath it. Simultaneously tap your right hand in sync with your foot. Feel the flow between your hand and foot, allowing that flow state to begin to resonate through your entire body. Allow this synchronised tapping to send a wave of relaxation through your entire system. Slowness is key here. Be sure to tap fewer than 60 taps per minute.

> Continue the process for around three minutes. If your mind wanders, that's perfectly normal; just redirect your focus back to the foot and hand tapping in unison.

> After three minutes add in a variation. Allow your right hand to settle and instead tap your left hand in sync with your right foot. After a few minutes allow your right foot to settle and allow your left foot to move in sync with your left hand. There are no hard and fast rules here. Play with the technique until you find your own rhythm and dance. Until you enter that flow-like state of mind.

> Notice how your mind becomes quieter in preparation for sleep.

For these techniques to work you only need three things: imagination, positive intent and intelligence. I truly believe if you are reading this you have already proved you have all three, so I see no reason why these will not work for you once you commit to trying them regularly until you see the results for yourself.

6

THE MAGIC OF THE BLACK BALLOON

While the last chapter dealt with soothing the mind, this one focuses on anxiety, and what you can do to combat it if it's interfering with your sleep.

You'll learn a technique that can help you with anxiety, and it's one of the nine Psychological Sleep Hacks you can choose from, in combination with your chosen Sleep Hacks from the Physical and Hypnomagical sections.

I'm fortunate enough to be able to control my anxiety levels, so they never become overwhelming. This is not because I'm just freakishly lucky, but because over the years I have trained myself to deal with my anxiety in different ways. I've been through a lot of research, and trial and error; and I have the tools I need at my disposal. I've learned to use these tools to mentally programme my mind to deal with anxiety regardless of external forces or circumstances. But I have huge empathy for people who struggle with anxiety, and it's something that people from all walks of life come to me looking for help with.

Anxiety affects people at different levels and in different ways. It's not just about people with a clinical diagnosis of an anxiety disorder. We live in an anxiety-inducing world, fuelled by everything from climate change to wars, the cost of living and more. Social media doesn't help either, as we look at pictures of other people's lives, which seem to be impossibly perfect, even though we know in our heart of hearts that they're just depicting their 'best possible' selves online. No one is immune from anxiety. Some people deal with anxiety in an instinctual manner; others with coping mechanisms, of which there are many, including but not limited to CBT (cognitive behavioural therapy), walking in nature, talk therapy, cold showers, ice baths, meditation, exercise, and more. Some people are lost in the noise of solutions, not knowing what to try or what to do. The good news is there is always a solution. You just need to commit to finding the one that works for you.

In this chapter, I'm introducing you to one of the most powerful techniques I use on both myself and my clients, a visualisation technique I call the Magic of the Black Balloon. The whole idea behind it is enabling you to let go of negative thought patterns in order to quieten the conscious mind and as a result become lighter in mind and body. It has had terrific results over the years.

Visualisation can help us create a new reality, and this is backed up by science. A 2015 study discovered something fascinating using a functional MRI (fMRI) machine to scan the participants' brain signals.[23] First, the participants viewed a piece of art while their brains were being scanned. Then they were asked to use visualisation techniques to imagine the piece of art that they had looked at. The brain signals were practically identical when they viewed the artwork compared with how they visualised the artwork. The brain did not perceive the difference between seeing the art versus imagining the art. That's a very compelling insight into why visualisation is so powerful.

A lot of sports stars use visualisation techniques, going right back to Muhammad Ali, who said, 'If my mind can conceive it, if my heart can believe it, then I can achieve it.' Footballer Wayne Rooney, tennis player Andy Murray and swimmer Michael Phelps use visualisation too.

Arnold Schwarzenegger credits visualisation for a lot of his success, first as a bodybuilder and then when he moved into acting and politics. The actor Jim Carrey is also a believer. Back in the early 1990s, his career wasn't exactly taking off. To motivate himself, he wrote himself a cheque for $10 million, dated 1994, for 'acting services rendered'. In 1994, he received $10 million for his starring role in *Dumb and Dumber*.

We can also learn a lot from Oprah Winfrey. More than any other celebrity, she has introduced the public to the power of visualisation. Born into poverty in rural Mississippi, she went on to achieve enormous success; at one point she was the world's only Black billionaire. She faced many challenges throughout her life but what kept her going throughout was her positive thinking, and visualisation. She noted, 'Create the highest, grandest vision possible for your life, because you become what you believe.'

All these examples are people who have used visualisation to pursue their dreams. But it's not only for people in search of success. It's regularly used as a technique to help people deal with anxiety. And anxiety is the enemy of sleep.

A different visualisation study looked at what happens to the brain when people visualise. Researchers asked subjects to imagine themselves somewhere in nature, or in a more urban setting, like a shopping centre or an apartment building.[24] As spending time in nature has been shown to reduce anxiety, the researchers wanted to see if this was the case if you simply visualised yourself being somewhere rural. The answer was yes: the brain processes visual imagery in the same way that it does actual experiences. In the study, 48 adults who had anxiety-like symptoms did 10-minute guided imagery sessions that were led by an audio recording. They were asked to visualise a natural or an urban scene of their choosing. They were also asked to make the experience more 'real' by visualising colours and shapes around them; engaging in other senses like touch and smell; and imagining themselves interacting with the scene. Before and after the sessions they filled out a questionnaire to measure their anxiety levels. The results showed that both the nature and the urban scenes reduced their anxiety, but the effect was more pronounced when nature imagery was used.

MEET TOM

Now I'd like to introduce you to Tom. Back during the recession, in 2009, I received an email from him through my website. He was from the northeast of the country, and was a very wealthy individual. To an ordinary observer he had everything. But unbeknownst to his family, friends and colleagues, the banks had taken his car, his house, all his assets, and he felt he had nothing left to live for. The gist of the email was:

> *I've tried everything to help myself out of this dark place and I'm writing this email as my last resort. I was about to take my life a few hours ago, and I'm giving myself a few hours. Only Keith Barry can help me. If he doesn't help me in the next few hours, I may indeed take my life.*

I felt a huge amount of pressure when I read that. I've helped thousands of ordinary people with everyday issues such as anxiety, stress, sleep, phobias and many more issues by using hypnosis as the tool, but I'm not without my failures. Some people simply don't respond to my suggestions, or for some reason I may not be able to connect with them on a deep psychological level.

Hypnosis relies on the relationship between the hypnotist and the client. That relationship is built on trust, faith, belief in the hypnotist, the language skills and experience of the hypnotist, and many more factors. It's not an exact science and it doesn't work on 100 per cent of people 100 per cent of the time. I'm reminded of the time I put on a 'stop smoking' seminar in Kildare in 2016. The event was an amazing success, with hundreds of people who successfully quit smoking. However, there were several disgruntled people who did not quit smoking. Some of these people decided to air their opinions in the press rather than contact us directly to allow us to assist them with their grievances. This resulted in a lot of negative pressure, and although people still contact me to this very day about the positive outcome that event had on their life, I decided to stop doing these 'stop smoking' events. I will say that it is unfortunate

I stopped, as although I would have undoubtedly failed with some people, I conservatively estimate that if I had kept doing them at least 1,500 people would have stopped smoking (based on one event per year over the past seven years).

I consistently approach every project with genuine intentions and a sincere commitment, so when anyone attacks my integrity it really does affect me. When I fail in a performance on stage or on a TV show, I learn quickly from the failure and then simply move on. But when I fail when attempting to help people, I find it super difficult on an emotional level and the feeling of failure can last for months.

Now that you have context, back to Tom. This is what went through my mind after thinking deeply about his email: 'If I decide not to help Tom and he kills himself I will have that on my conscience for the rest of my life. Conversely, if I do attempt to help him but it doesn't work, and he kills himself, I will have that on my conscience for the rest of my life.' It was a lose–lose situation unless I could help him dramatically improve his mental health. After considering all this carefully, I decided I would do what I could to help him.

Tom came to a large venue in Cork where I was playing. He came to my dressing room and I went through the process of how to release conscious problems and anxieties with the Magic of the Black Balloon. I asked him to commit wholeheartedly that he would use the technique every single night before he attempted to go to sleep. You see, Tom was hugely sleep-deprived. The level of anxiety that he had from his mounting problems was interfering greatly with his sleep. Some nights he would procrastinate for so many hours he would end up falling asleep at 4 a.m. and waking up again by 6 a.m.

Other nights he would fall asleep by 1 a.m. but wake within an hour! His anxiety was feeding his lack of sleep and his lack of sleep was feeding his anxiety. He felt trapped in a continuous negative loop where he was finding it hard to simply even exist. We'll get back to Tom a little later.

What happens to you when you feel anxious? Your limbic system, known as 'the emotional brain', comprises your hypothalamus, hippocampus and amygdala. They all have fascinating roles to play. The hypothalamus is what helps our body maintain a steady internal state; it controls autonomic functions like hunger, thirst and body temperature. Meanwhile, the hippocampus is where our memories are created and stored, and is also responsible for spatial memory and navigation. Then there's the amygdala, which is of most interest to us in this context, because it's the control centre of the nervous system and is what causes us to react when we are in a dangerous or potentially dangerous situation. It's a tiny, almond-shaped part of the brain, but it has a huge impact on how we behave as it's also responsible for feelings like anger, fear and happiness. There's something called the amygdala 'hijack', where the amygdala is overwhelmed by stress, and even though there is no physical danger present, it takes over the brain and the person isn't able to make a rational response. Research indicates that a hyperactive amygdala is associated with anxiety disorders, panic attacks, obsessive-compulsive disorder, and depression.[25]

Simply put, when the limbic system is activated in a stressful situation, the stress hormones adrenaline, noradrenaline and cortisol are released into our body. Unless we have a method to release or relieve the effects of these chemicals, our bodies will go into overload mode, which results in the feeling that is known as anxiety.

FLIGHT OR FIGHT

It reminds me of a time I went to a friend's house when I was 16. Tammy Holman had a large German shepherd dog called Lady which she had rescued when she was abandoned as a pup and found tied to a tree. We were chatting outside Tammy's house in Ballygunner, Waterford, when Lady began to show her teeth and growl. I said to Tammy I thought Lady was about to attack. She smiled and said Lady had never attacked anyone. Then I saw the dog's lips peel all the way back to show her gums, and in that instant I knew she was 100 per cent about to attack. My legs went to jelly as my limbic system fired up. Fear pulsed through every atom in my body. For a moment I froze with the rush of chemicals pulsing through my system. And then I ran. I ran like Usain Bolt on 40 cups of coffee for the 3-foot wall at the top of Tammy's garden. As I was running I could hear Lady's teeth chomping behind my backside. I jumped the wall and amazingly Lady stopped. I guess she didn't take kindly to a brain hacker, but luckily for me she was just protecting the perimeter of her property. Immediately the fight or flight symptoms began to release their grip on me as Tammy sheepishly walked my mountain bike down to me and I cycled home, none the worse for the experience. This experience shows how useful the limbic system can be, but also how powerful an effect it can have over both our mind and our body.

Weirdly, I am reminded of another experience on the same road where Tammy lives, but this time with a more negative consequence.

My granddad on my mother's side was known as Gaga. This dated from the time my sister couldn't pronounce 'Granddad' so she started calling him Gaga instead, and then I and all my cousins called him Gaga right into adulthood. Gaga told me this story from when he was young, sometime in the 1940s. He and a few of his friends decided to play a prank on another guy, who used to cycle to work every morning at about 5 a.m. We're talking about a dark, lonely country road.

The prank was that Gaga lay down in a field and his two friends lit lots of candles around him and they hid in a ditch. Back in those days, if you saw that, you'd wonder, is that a ghost? Is it a cult? Is it an alien? You wouldn't really know what you were looking at. This guy was cycling along and he stopped on his bike and he let out a shriek of fear, and then he just cycled off as fast as he could. The lads, of course, thought this was hilarious. The sad part about the story is that the guy on the bike never spoke another word for the rest of his life. The prank that turned so horribly wrong shows the physiological response that we can have to fear, and sometimes these reactions can be uncontrollable. This true story illustrates the physiological reactions we universally experience in response to fear, and shows that at times our responses can be beyond our control.

I've presented two extreme examples here, but they're crucial in highlighting the influence of the subconscious response, specifically the limbic system in action, and its relationship with the conscious mind.

In the third section of this book I will share some tools to hack your subconscious mind to achieve deep sleep, but what if I told you that you have the power to hack your conscious mind to control your anxieties? Your mind is the world's first supercomputer and you have the ability to input, extract and even erase information, both consciously and subconsciously, if you have the correct tools and toolkit.

TRY THIS: TRIANGLE BREATHING TO REDUCE ANXIETY This breathing system is designed to reduce anxiety and induce relaxation by regulating your breathing in a triangular pattern.

> - Inhale for three seconds. Start by taking a long, deep breath in through your nose as you count to three in your mind.
> - Exhale for three seconds. Be sure to exhale slowly and completely through your mouth.
> - Pause for three seconds. Simply stop breathing for a count of three before starting the cycle again.

Repeat the triangular breathing system for a number of rounds, adjusting the timelines based on your comfort level. The key is to enter into a flow state and ensure each phase of breathing lasts for an equal length of time, creating a triangular pattern.

HACKING YOUR CONSCIOUS MIND

Until the late twentieth century, the science said that once we were in our teens or early twenties, our brains were fully formed and couldn't be changed. However, we now know that is completely untrue and that our brain is shifting and changing all the time. Neuroplasticity, as it's known, means that many aspects of the brain can be altered, or are 'plastic'. In fact, it's ongoing throughout life; neuroplasticity never stops. You can shape-shift your brain all the way into your seventies, eighties and nineties. We have, on average, 86 billion neurons in our brain, and we're creating new neural pathways every second of every day. You are not the same person now that you were ten seconds ago, and in another ten seconds you won't be the person you are right now. If you stop and think about it, you will acknowledge that you're not the same person you were five years ago, and that change has happened over time. Every second and every thought you create counts!

This is why the Magic of the Black Balloon is amazing. It allows you to change and shape-shift your brain to create a new reality for yourself and help eliminate negative thoughts.

Imagine your brain is like a lump of clay, or a lump of marla plasticine, as I knew it back in the day. You can stretch and alter your brain using the Magic of the Black Balloon, transforming its capabilities. Keep in mind that your brain is flexible, and it's crucial to engage and exercise it just like you would your physical body. Exercising your mind for good brain health can also help optimise your sleep.

To keep my brain healthy, I do everything from Rubik's cubes to puzzles to writing to reading. I do a lot of different things, but the one thing I recommend every single person does is visualisation, both consciously and subconsciously.

Brain fitness has all kinds of benefits and it's never too late to start doing a brain workout. The key is to find something that offers novelty and challenge. That could be driving a different way home, doing a Sudoku, learning a new language, writing with your non-dominant hand, or getting creative at dinner time and trying something new. A study published in 2020 found that regularly shaking up your routine and doing a diverse array of activities throughout adulthood can boost cognitive functioning and decelerate the signs of ageing like memory loss and declining information processing.[26]

Neuroplasticity means that you can work through your anxiety, and with enough repetition you can create a new neural pathway to create a buffer between the cause of anxiety and your response. It's about changing the script and telling yourself a different story.

Essentially, we all have busy minds and anxieties and fears, and we need to alleviate those in order to promote good sleep.

SLEEP HACK 13
THE MAGIC OF THE BLACK BALLOON

An audio recording where I guide you through this visualisation can be accessed on my website www.keithbarry.com/sleephacks with the password SLEEPHACKS24.

The Magic of the Black Balloon works to reduce those negative thoughts and here's how to do it:

- Start by closing your eyes.
- Now imagine that there is a hole in the very top of your head and attached to that hole is a deflated black balloon.
- As you lie comfortably and quietly in your bed, allow yourself to feel the feelings of any anxiety you have, in your body or in your mind. Perhaps you feel it in your head or chest, or maybe you feel it in your breathing, or in some part of your brain. Just allow that moment of anxiety to be there and lie with it for a minute. Now, focus on that anxiety and where exactly it is in your body. If it's in your head, try and find the position in your head – is it the front, the right-hand side or the back? Is it tension in your neck? Is it a feeling in your chest? Is it a sick feeling in your stomach? Locate wherever that anxiety is in your body.

- Now visualise and imagine that point of anxiety moving from where it is up and all the way to the very top of your head. Imagine that you're bringing that thought, that sensation, and releasing it into the black balloon. Now find another negative thought or anxiety or fear, and visualise that going into the black balloon. Every worry, every fear, and now all of them are entering and inflating the black balloon. The big worries, the tiny ones, the work deadline you have tomorrow; getting the kids' lunch ready in a hurry; your concerns about money; your relationship worries; any negative thoughts – they are all being funnelled into the black balloon.
- With every problem or issue you send into the balloon, imagine that black balloon inflating bigger and bigger and bigger and bigger and bigger, up over your head, so big that it's almost ready to burst. It's only just ready to burst when you are sure it's completely filled with all the negative thoughts, emotions, questions and words that are troubling you. Just let all of them go into the black balloon.
- As you do that, now imagine that you reach up to your head and you just quickly tie off the balloon. Now, the moment you have that knot tied and you have that black balloon filled with your anxieties and fears and thoughts, let go of the balloon. It starts to rise, slowly at first, floating away from you.
- In your mind you see the black balloon floating out of an imaginary open window. You look through the window and up at that black balloon as it floats higher and higher and higher. But as it ascends into the sky, into the distance, you notice that it begins to get smaller and smaller. As it gets

smaller and smaller, you notice it gets less and less significant as it goes up and up and up away into the vast sky. Perhaps it's floating over your neighbour's house or maybe it's being blown so far into the distance you can barely see it. You see it one last time before it dissipates and disappears, and then you immediately find that you're left with a sense of calmness, a sense of relief, a sense of serenity. Just allow yourself to sit with that for a moment.

> Now that the balloon is gone, and now that you've just allowed yourself to sit with that calmness, notice a sense of solitude you find inside yourself.

> Find again that place inside yourself where you felt that first thought of anxiety or depression or unhappiness. Find that spot and now begin to fill that spot with radiant, purple light. That exact place where you initially found the disruptive feeling is now filled with purple light that brings you self-assurance, calmness, positivity. You find that calming sensation spreading out through your whole body, glowing internally, and that positivity, that calmness, spreads into every muscle, nerve and fibre of your physical body.

> Once that happens, to finish, I want you to silently repeat the following five times, in preparation for sleep:
I am free from my anxieties and fears
I release what no longer serves me
I embrace a light and peaceful mind, ready for bed.

Read the Magic of the Black Balloon at least three times, and at the end of the chapter you can find a quick recap on your key action points for this.

A NOTE ON AFFIRMATIONS

Throughout the book, as part of different techniques, I've included affirmations. If you're not familiar with what they are, these are short, positive statements that have a particular meaning for you. The first time I discovered an affirmation was when I was in my early teens and read an affirmation by French psychologist and pharmacist Émile Coué, who coined the phrase: 'Every day in every way, I am getting better and better.' I would say this to myself every single morning before I went to school and every single night before I went to bed. This had a profound effect on my psyche. If you repeat something over and over so that it enters the subconscious you will notice that real magic can happen. This is classic auto-suggestion, as developed by Coué at the beginning of the twentieth century. He wrote, 'If you persuade yourself that you can do a certain thing, provided this thing be possible, you will do it, however difficult it may be. If, on the contrary, you imagine that you cannot do the simplest thing in the world, it is impossible for you to do it, and molehills become for you unscalable mountains.'

If you're on social media, you're probably very aware of how popular self-affirmations are, because the internet is packed with them. Indeed, they frequently become the target of ridicule and various forms of criticism, with the underlying idea behind this humour being that if positive thinking could resolve every issue, all problems would cease to exist. Although all those perfect-looking Instagrammers posting motivational messaging can sometimes seem disingenuous and self-serving, it's not a reason to not utilise positive affirmations, because the science behind them is solid.

Numerous studies have shown that there's a lot of power in

self-affirmations, and that they can improve your health and your wellbeing in many ways. One study showed that self-affirmations help to change behaviours around health. It found that self-affirmations encouraged people to eat significantly more fruit and vegetables over a two-week period than those who didn't self-affirm.[27] Additional research revealed that individuals who use smartphones excessively and engage in self-affirmation experience a notable reduction in phone usage of 57.2 per cent.[28] Furthermore, fMRI studies demonstrate that self-affirmation stimulates the brain's reward system, a region associated with pleasure.[29]

Affirmations work best when they align with your core values and what you truly believe in, and what you believe about yourself, and what you believe is possible. You'll note that I'm not giving you affirmations such as *I am going to fall asleep immediately.*

I could potentially use trance work or hypnosis to help you fall asleep immediately if you were sitting right in front of me, and that's because I have studied the skill for years. But to help you fall asleep and to feel confident that you can do so, I'm giving you gentle affirmations that you know are within your capabilities.

The affirmations I'm giving you are believable and achievable, so there's no pressure in feeling they're something you can't do; they're all possible.

An affirmation has to be:

> Something meaningful to you
> Something that is specific
> Something that is credible and possible within reason
> Something that is deeply personal
> Something that you practise on a daily/nightly basis

- Something that focuses on a positive goal instead of the negative (e.g. *I am ready to embrace a restful sleep* versus *I don't want to wake up during the night*)
- Something that is said in the present tense
- Something that you are committed to – in this case, achieving a restful and restorative night's sleep, because you have identified how important this is for your wellbeing.

Of those points above, the really important one to note is that affirmations are said in the present tense and you really allow yourself to believe that it's already happened. In other words, if you want to feel better, say it in the now and allow it to become your new reality, allowing your mind to think that it's real. Over time, through repetition, the idea, the affirmation, will become fact.

Self-affirmations are not a magic bullet, but then again, nothing is. But if you use them as part of the techniques in this book, and if you practise them, they will help you on your sleep journey and can be life-enhancing.

A simple but amazingly effective affirmation is an ancient one use by Hawaiian people called Ho'oponopono, which translates roughly as 'cause things to move back in balance'. It's both a healing practice and a prayer that offers reconciliation and forgiveness. A four-line mantra, Ho'oponopono consists of the following words:

I'm Sorry, Forgive Me, Thank You, I Love You.

'I'm Sorry' is about admitting responsibility for whatever issue is in your life, and feeling remorse for having caused it.

'Forgive Me' can be both self-forgiveness and directed towards other people, and this is a necessary cleansing step in the ritual.

'Thank You' is where you express gratitude for all that you are, all that you have, all that you are part of and all that will become.

'I Love You' allows you to send healing waves of love to your body, yourself and your surroundings, and to let yourself feel imbued with the positive energy of this feeling.

I use lots of different affirmations to achieve different outcomes in my own life. Every time I get in my ice bath, I repeat over and over: *I am happy. I am healthy. I am resilient.* When I am in a cold shower, I repeat: *I control this mind. I control this body. No one controls this mind or body but me.* When I am using the Black Balloon I will use: *I am free from my anxieties and fears, I release what no longer serves me, I embrace a light and peaceful mind, ready for bed.* But sometimes I will change or switch this up by saying something else such as: *I deserve this sleep. I will recover tonight. Tomorrow will be an amazing day.*

There really is no hard or fast rule when it comes to affirmations. Be creative and jot some down right now that you believe will help you. Here are a few examples to get you started.

TRY THIS: PICK ONE OF THESE AFFIRMATIONS AND USE IT FOR A MONTH

- Tonight is the night my sleep improves by at least one per cent.
- Every day in every way my sleep will get better and better.
- With every breath I embrace rest and reduce stress and my sleep progresses.
- Achieving a good night's sleep is my new norm.
- Nothing and no one will interfere with my sleep tonight.

'What about Tom?' I hear you ask. Tom found the technique enormously helpful. All these years later, he still sends me postcards on occasion from various places he goes to all over the world just to say thanks for releasing his anxieties. He's enjoying life's pleasures and enjoying being infinitely curious about the world, and although he's not as wealthy now as he used to be he's wealthy in his mind. That's how effective the Magic of the Black Balloon can be, and it can be used just as successfully to lead you towards a tranquil sleep.

THE MAGIC OF THE BLACK BALLOON: SIX THINGS TO REMEMBER

1. Imagine there is a hole at the top of your head.
2. Locate where the anxiety is in your body, and sit with it.
3. Visualise that anxiety or negative thought or stressful feeling travel to the top of your head, slowly filling the balloon.
4. Continue to fill the black balloon until it is almost bursting, then tie a knot and let it go.
5. As it floats away and becomes insignificant, imagine a purple radiant light spreading through the spot in your body where the tension was previously located.
6. Repeat your affirmation and prepare for sleep.

The Magic of the Black Balloon is an exceptionally powerful technique and I am confident that you can harness its potency.

7

MIND WIPE

In this, the final chapter in the Psychological section, I am introducing you to the final two Sleep Hacks in this section, Hacks 14 and 15 – and once again reminding you that you can choose any one of the Sleep Hacks 7–15 from this section. To begin, I'd like to tell you about a young man who turned his life around with the technique in this chapter.

MEET PATRICK

Back in 2004 in the fast-paced world of motivational speaking, at the age of 28, Patrick was a fresh-faced, relatively unknown newcomer to the industry.

He stood out as an entertaining, inspiring and passionate speaker, with an ability to inspire and motivate audiences and attendees at events where he was booked to perform. However, his constant pursuit of perfection regularly took a toll on his much-needed rest.

As he prepared for a crucial speaking engagement, Patrick found himself fully immersed in meticulously preparing his presentation. Late nights became a regular occurrence as he tirelessly prepared his PowerPoint presentation, driven by a constant flow of caffeine and the drive to deliver an unforgettable and memorable performance. He snacked into the late hours, sacrificing his usual bedtime routine in the name of perfecting his presentation.

When he finally did manage to hit the hay, Patrick continued to rehearse his speech over and over in his mind and mulled over what might go wrong. He thought to himself: 'Will I flub a line? Will the audience heckle me? What if the microphone doesn't work? What if I faint? What if I trip walking out? What if no one applauds?' Overwhelmed by the pressure to perfect his presentation, he struggled with his sleep patterns, tossing and turning as he overthought every aspect of the presentation. The stress of it all stopped him falling asleep for up to two hours after his head hit the pillow.

The night before his presentation, after just two hours of light sleep, Patrick awoke at 5 a.m. as if he had had a nightmare. Strangely enough, he didn't remember any dreams or nightmares at all. He just had that nightmarish jolt which woke him up as if he had seen a ghost. Instead of staying in bed for some much-needed rest and recuperation, he gave in to the urge to open the laptop in bed and return to his PowerPoint, prolonging the cycle of sleep deprivation. After a while he threw the laptop aside and began to snooze again. The soundtrack of *The A-Team* (his chosen alarm sound) signified the beginning of yet another challenging day, and despite actually now needing to get up and prepare for the day ahead, he whacked the snooze button, exhausted from the challenges of a night's broken sleep.

His presentation received a mixed response due to a somewhat lacklustre performance. Patrick's tiredness manifested in him forgetting his script. His presentation was packed with filler words and lacked his usual dynamic energy. Although he considered the performance acceptable, the effects of lack of sleep on his wellbeing were apparent during his speech. Unbeknownst to him, the consequence of sleep deprivation showed on the stage during his performance and was also impacting his overall health and effectiveness.

After his presentation, Patrick opted to unwind and reward himself for his hard work by going to the pub, ignoring the persistent ill effects the restless nights were having on his mental and physical health. Little did he realise that unless he changed his sleep habits, his sleep-deprived state would have implications beyond the immediate aftermath of the presentation, and would negatively impact his overall health and long-term wellbeing.

However, that night, his mum sat him down and gave it to him straight. 'Son, you look terrible. You're only 25 but already look 40. You've got a double chin and dark rings under your eyes and I'm scared. I'm scared I'll have to sing at your funeral.'

Patrick was shocked. He had no idea just how big a toll the lack of sleep had taken on him. Recognising it was a problem, but Patrick promised his mum that he would attempt to prioritise his sleep and harness the power of a well-rested mind. He told his mother that he would do whatever it took.

Patrick began by targeting good sleep hygiene. He established a consistent sleep schedule, which allowed his body to harmonise with its natural circadian rhythm. He created a healthy and calm night-time routine, incorporating relaxing activities and eliminating screen time before his head hit the pillow. Patrick also remodelled his entire bedroom – he installed blackout curtains, a humidifier and a Himalayan salt lamp, ensuring it was a space conducive to relaxation and serenity.

However, the true transformational moment came when Patrick discovered my Mind Wipe technique, a powerful psychological tool for silencing the constant inner voice of his hyperactive mind. This technique involves an intentional process of recognising and releasing racing thoughts, allowing the mind to quieten in preparation for sleep.

As Patrick committed to these changes, over a number of weeks the changes were extraordinary. His energy levels skyrocketed, and a newfound clarity penetrated every aspect of his life. The real test, however, came out of the blue when he was invited to deliver a talk at the prestigious TED conference. The TED platform is known globally as a premier stage for global thought leaders, performers, visionaries and creatives, where they can share ground-breaking thoughts and concepts. This was by far Patrick's biggest break to date and not one where he would want a repeat of the performance mentioned in the previous paragraphs.

Armed with a solid foundation of sleep, which was catalysed by using my Mind Wipe technique, Patrick took to the stage with a new sense of confidence, one he hadn't felt before. His words flowed effortlessly, his energy was contagious and his dynamic presence captivated the audience, who gave him a standing ovation. The impact was immense and immediate – his TED talk resonated with people on a global scale.

His presentation went viral, capturing the attention of millions and earning Patrick a spot among the top 20 TED talks of all time.

The longevity of its influence was unprecedented, remaining in the top tier of TED's most-viewed talks for an astonishing 20 years.

Patrick's journey illustrates that true success isn't just about putting in the hours, slogging it out and working hard; it is about looking after one's wellbeing, understanding the correlation between good sleep and performance, and unlocking the potential of a rested mind.

SILENCING YOUR NOISY THOUGHTS

Do you ever feel your brain's fizzing? You have so many thoughts stirring around that it feels as if your mind might either explode or implode. Most of us have experienced that inner voice, keeping us awake as we lie in bed. It's like having an ice cream machine or a washing machine buzzing away, keeping you from the sleep that you crave.

We often have many ideas bouncing around, some of them important, others less relevant, as we try to sleep. Here are a few ideas my Instagram audience answered in response to a questionnaire I posted asking them, 'What kind of silly thoughts keep you awake as you attempt to sleep?'

> *Did I lock the back door?*
> *What if my alarm doesn't go off tomorrow?*
> *I'm not ready for the big meeting on Friday!*
> *Why did I arrange to meet someone after work when I'd rather go home to my couch?*
> *I think that person took what I said the wrong way.*
> *I keep buying clothes I don't need and my credit card bill is terrifying.*

> *What will I cook for dinner tomorrow?*
> *Will my mother remember she has the kids after school?*
> *Can I skip the gym tomorrow?*
> *How can I quit my job?*
> *Why is the pain in my shoulder getting worse?*
> *The house is a tip and I don't have the energy to sort it out.*
> *I'm so annoyed my boss called a meeting for 4.30 p.m.*
> *Can polystyrene go in the recycling bin? Better check.*
> *How am I going to be able to afford a holiday this year?*
> *I forgot to text my sister back and she's going to be annoyed.*

And so it goes, on and on and on. These are examples of everyday anxieties that niggle at a lot of people as they lie in bed. We're not talking here about people who suffer anxiety disorders, or major life events that can cause stress, like divorce, or the loss of a loved one, or job loss or chronic illness. Nope, it's the annoying and invasive thoughts that are taking up real estate in your head, but that shouldn't warrant you sacrificing healing and restorative sleep to think about them.

I've mentioned this in an earlier chapter – the Buddhist concept of the monkey mind, where you feel confused and unsettled due to the constant stream of unwanted or random thoughts, uncontrollably jumping from one thought to another and another and another. These thoughts can often include fantasies, concepts, plans for the next day, and problems from the previous day, worries, concerns and random weird images that distract from the task at hand – SLEEP!

I often refer to these thoughts as the busy bees – everything is buzzing around and making a noise in your head just like bees moving from one flower to another. Your mind is speeding, racing and buzzing, but all you want to do is go to sleep. This overwhelming influx of concerns, ideas and emotions can play a significant factor in keeping you awake when all you really want to do is go to sleep. Even when you are physically exhausted and consciously ready for bed these thoughts can keep you awake for hours and hours. When your brain is filled with concerns and ideas it finds it difficult to calm down when it really should be transitioning into a restful state. The good news is that you can learn to train your mind to settle down these busy thoughts. But first you need a basic understanding of what is happening inside your brain.

The prefrontal cortex, which is that part of your brain associated with regulating your thoughts, actions and decisions, begins to activate instead of winding down. During the day this region of the brain is heavily engaged in various cognitive tasks such as planning and goal-orientated behaviour.

The issue arises when night falls and the prefrontal cortex doesn't switch off as quickly as desired. When the busy thoughts about the day you've just had or the day you're about to have come into play, this only magnifies the intensity of these fizzy thoughts.

When that happens, many people get so stressed about their inability to sleep that they develop sleep anxiety, which can also prevent you from entering deep sleep and can cause you to wake during the night. Sleep anxiety is a form of performance anxiety, where you begin to feel stressed about your ability to perform a certain task. It can lead to sleep deprivation, which could mean that you get caught up in the infinity sleep deprivation loop. This perpetual cycle of a racing mind coupled with anxiety creates a detrimental loop which needs to be eliminated using a calm and centred approach.

There is another part of the brain called the reticular activating system (RAS), a complex network of neurons located in the brainstem, which plays a crucial role in alertness, wakefulness and concentration. It acts as a filter for incoming sensory information, determining which stimuli are relevant and should be brought to conscious attention. The RAS is intimately involved in the regulation of the sleep–wake cycle. During wakefulness, the RAS is more active, promoting alertness and responsiveness to stimuli. When someone begins to transition into sleep, the RAS should naturally decrease, allowing other sleep-promoting mechanisms to take over.

When someone is getting ready for sleep, there should be a reduction in RAS activity, which in turn triggers a series of other physiological processes leading to relaxation of the mind and the body, making it easier to transition into sleep. When the RAS reduces its activity during the onset of sleep, other neurotransmitter systems such as melatonin become more active.

If the RAS does not begin to shut down at night for some reason, this can contribute to various sleep-related issues. For instance, if the RAS remains overly active, it can result in difficulties falling or staying asleep, contributing to insomnia. Conversely, if the RAS is underactive during wakeful hours, it may lead to excessive drowsiness during the daytime.

External factors such as stress, nervousness, tension, and certain medications can influence the activity of the RAS. Chronic stress, for example, may lead to prolonged activation of the RAS, disrupting the balance between wakefulness and sleep.

Understanding the intimate relationship between the RAS and the sleep cycle provides insights into the complexity of sleep processes. It emphasises the need for a holistic approach to sleep hygiene, including stress management and lifestyle choices, to support the proper functioning of the RAS and promote healthy sleep patterns.

The busy bees and noisy thoughts at night keep both the RAS and the prefrontal cortex activated. However, as a brain hacker I'm about to share with you methods of hacking your own brain to quell these thoughts and in turn settle these parts of your brain in preparation for a good night's rest.

TRY THIS: MAKE A MEMORY SCENT JAR TO CALM A BUSY MIND

> Take some time to remember some times when you were peaceful and at your happiest.
> Notice what smells were present in these memories. Perhaps the smell of flowers, leather, freshly baked bread – any smells at all that you can remember.
> Get a jar with a lid and over the coming days gather some items which have a smell similar to the smells in your memories. Try to find non-perishable items such as sachets of herbs, dried flowers or aromatic spices.
> Arrange the items thoughtfully in the jar to ensure visual appeal.
> If you want to intensify the smell add some drops of essential oils that match your memories most closely.
> Seal the jar and label it with the date of the memory and the name of the location where it took place.
> When you need to calm your busy mind, open the jar, close your eyes, inhale and allow the scent to invoke the calming memories that come to mind.

Decide right now to adopt the methods outlined in the next few pages to empty and erase these noisy thoughts which will naturally then soothe and comfort your mind in preparation for sleep.

Note that this isn't necessarily about alleviating anxiety and stress. That is something I've already shown you how to achieve in the Magic of the Black Balloon chapter. This Mind Wipe technique is designed to help you stop your internal hamster-on-a-wheel and busy bee voices in your mind and help you deal with overthinking about everything from work to studying for exams to your plans for tomorrow.

Throughout the years, I have performed thousands of Mind Wipes, where I have erased someone's whole memory of who they are and what they are. Every thought they have had, every word they have uttered, even the memory of their own name is just gone. It might look unbelievable, but anybody who has seen me at one of my countless live shows can attest to me being able to do this to random strangers.

One of my favourite experiences ever of doing a Mind Wipe was filmed for my show on the Discovery Channel. It took place at the War Memorial in Michigan. I met a guy called Christophe, his friend who had known him since kindergarten, and Christophe's girlfriend. I asked Christophe if it would be okay if I tried a little experiment with him. He agreed.

I started by explaining that there are two different types of memory. There's long-term memory, which is where everything that we've ever experienced is stored. Then there's short-term memory, which is where we store memories like where we put our keys (but a few moments later we might not be able to remember where we've put them).

Then I told Christophe that I wanted to access that part of his memory where all his files are stored, right behind the ears, an area called the temporal lobe. I instructed him to bring up all those memories – every single memory from his life up and across and down and into his forehead, into the frontal lobe.

After that, using black ops hypnosis, I informed him I was erasing every single memory from his mind – going, going, gone! I asked him if he recognised the people with him – his childhood friend and his girlfriend. He didn't. He didn't know where he was. I handed him a mirror and asked him if he recognised the face looking back at him – and amazingly he didn't!

This looked miraculous to the untrained eye, the muggles, as we friendly hypnotists refer to you, the viewers. However, I can assure you this was not a miracle of any kind. I had simply put Christophe into a waking trance where I could then use my secret RSVP technique to eliminate his entire life from his mind. A Mind Wipe if you will. What does RSVP stand for? Rhythm, Speed, Volume and Pitch. By changing all four aspects of my voice in a very specific way, I have the ability to hypnotise people through conversational hypnosis, beneath their cognitive level of awareness.

After bringing him out of his hypnotic state, he was able to say his name was Christophe, he knew the date, and he knew he was with his best friend and his girlfriend. I restored him back to his normal self with no harm done, although he had no memory of what just took place. When his two companions told him what had happened, he couldn't believe it. But it was there, recorded on camera for posterity, and you can still find the clip on YouTube.

Why was this one of my favourite Mind Wipes? The true miracle actually occurred off camera and was never aired. In truth, I found the Christophe experience really interesting, but not because of the Mind Wipe technique I used on him. For the Discovery Channel show, we never knew any of the people we filmed beforehand, because we would randomly approach them on the street. But I discovered later, when the cameras stopped, that Christophe had always had a really bad stutter. I asked him if he would like me to use hypnosis to attempt to help him with his stutter. He agreed. I did an instant hypnotic stutter management technique there and then, never having assisted someone with a stutter in my life. Moments later the words flowed out of his mouth, like a stream of uninterrupted thoughts, carrying with them a new-found fluency and confidence that completely transformed the way he communicated. His friends lost their minds in disbelief, and even he was freaking out because he was now speaking so fluently and eloquently. I'd love to know how he's doing now, and it would be amazing if his stutter had diminished or disappeared for good.

But now, on to the techniques that will help you to calm your mind and rid yourself of those annoying, busy bee thoughts.

Although you won't be able to wipe your entire mind instantaneously (and it's not something I would recommend anyway!), you can still use a similar mind wiping technique on yourself in preparation for sleep. This works by giving the monkey mind something other than your own thoughts to focus on and then erasing even those focused thoughts down to nothing, so nothing exists in your mind except emptiness – a provision of space to induce a trance state towards slumber.

Below, you'll find my primary Mind Wipe technique, and this is the one that I'd like you to try first, while you're lying in bed. The other technique, the Galactic Mind Wipe, is a variation on that, which you might like to try once you've mastered the original Mind Wipe – especially if you like stars!

SLEEP HACK 14
MIND WIPE

An audio recording where I guide you through this visualisation can be accessed on my website www.keithbarry.com/sleephacks with the password SLEEPHACKS24.

> Lie on your bed, close your eyes and imagine that you are in a room that has nothing else in it. The room has four white walls, a white ceiling and a white floor. All the walls are wipeable whiteboards with a shiny surface, the kind you might see in any classroom or lecture hall.

> On each of the four walls you notice the word ALERT written in thick black jumbo erasable marker. The only person in the room is you, and you are also dressed all in white.

> I want you to imagine walking up to one of the whiteboards. As you walk towards it you can clearly see the word ALERT is written so big that it covers the entire whiteboard, but you also notice it is written inside a black dry-erase rectangle that borders the whiteboard.

> Now, in your mind, you walk up to that whiteboard, and you look at the word ALERT. You decide it's not a word that has any relevance at this moment, so you want to get rid of it. You notice a teeny tiny eraser on the whiteboard's ledge. The

smallest eraser you've ever seen. It's so small it's barely larger than a grain of rice. You pick it up and you realise that you must erase the word ALERT and the rectangle from the whiteboard. The only rule is you must use the eraser and nothing else. You mustn't even get any marker on your fingertips.

> Begin by carefully erasing the rectangle around the word ALERT. You slowly and diligently erase the entire rectangle. This should take a few minutes. Now, you begin to erase the word ALERT, starting with the T and working backwards. You notice how long it takes you to erase the word and you keep rubbing, rubbing, rubbing, rubbing, rubbing, rubbing, rubbing, rubbing. As you do this, remember to do it in real time with that tiny eraser. Eventually, after several minutes, the word ALERT is gone, erased.

> Once you have erased it from the first wall you know you must now erase the words and borders from the other three walls. Take your time to do this. If your mind wanders from this task, remind yourself to come back to the white room and to continue erasing the words until they are completely gone and the whiteboards are fully clear.

> When you have cleared all four whiteboards, allow yourself to imagine hearing a noise in the background. It's a very gentle and low-level static noise. It's white noise, as befits the white room, and it sounds like 'zzzzzzzzzzzzzz'.

> Now you notice that there's also a black marker on one of the whiteboard's ledges. It's a tiny, fine-point black marker. You are now going to use this marker to fill the whiteboard with the only word that has any significance right now. That word is, of course, SLEEP.

> Begin at the top left of the whiteboard and write out the word 'sleep' in lower case. And then keep writing the word 'sleep' until that whiteboard is full. It will take hundreds, if not thousands, of times writing the word to fill the whiteboard. Your only job at this moment is to do that task in your mind and keep writing the word 'sleep' until that whiteboard is full. It is the only task in your life that has any relevance right now.
> If you manage to fill one whiteboard without falling asleep, move on to the next one, and so on.
> If your mind wanders to any other thought as you're doing this in your imagination, remind yourself to come back to the process of being in the white room and writing out the word 'sleep'.

I have personally never encountered anyone who, if they use this process correctly, has successfully managed to fill all four whiteboards before they begin to doze off. But of course, you might be different. You might be that special person who for some reason just can't drift off. If that's you:

> Take the eraser again, but this time take it to all those thousands of words of sleep that you've written down and you begin to erase those, one letter at a time, backwards from the last p of the last s-l-e-e-p. Erase those words, one letter at a time.
> If you somehow manage to rewind all the way back to when the whiteboards are clean again and you are still not ready to settle into a deep and restorative sleep, take the black marker

again and start the process of filling the whiteboard all over again with the word 'sleep', doing so in real time. Repeat the process over and over until you actually do drift away.

The next hack is ideal for stargazers or even *Star Wars* fans!

SLEEP HACK 15
GALACTIC MIND WIPE

An audio recording where I guide you through this visualisation can be accessed on my website www.keithbarry.com/sleephacks with the password SLEEPHACKS24.

> Lie down, close your eyes and visualise the canvas of your mind as a gigantic galaxy containing thousands of stars of various sizes and intensities inside your mind. Every star symbolises a different worry, memory, thought, idea or concern that occupies your consciousness. Imagine these stars shimmering brightly against the vast backdrop of space itself.
> Take a moment to notice which stars are shining the brightest and acknowledge these stars individually. Perhaps there are ten of them shining brightly. Maybe more. Maybe less. You decide. You are in control of the galaxy and therefore in control of your monkey mind. Assign a specific worry or concern to each one. See the disruptive thought printed across the star itself. As you do this, observe the constellation of your thoughts, recognising the variety of concerns that have become busy bees or manic monkeys in your mind.

> Now, one by one, visualise these stars beginning to transform into shooting stars. As each disruptive thought or worry morphs into a streak of light, imagine it gracefully fading away, disappearing into the distance, leaving only the calming and soothing glow of the remaining stars in the galaxy. Begin to observe a calmness and stillness now in your new mental cosmic universe. Continue to do this until all the brightest stars have vanished
> Embrace tranquillity. Mentally bathe in the gentle comfort of your new mental galaxy, completely free from the intensity of intrusive thoughts. The shooting stars have carried away your busy bees and chaotic monkeys, leaving behind a peaceful cosmic landscape. Feel the weight of your worries dissipate and disappear as you prepare to drift into a tranquil and restful sleep.

By visualising your concerns as stars in a galaxy and allowing them to transform into shooting stars, you are creating a calming rewiring of the brain that facilitates the transition from a cluttered mind to a state of serenity, paving the way for a peaceful night's sleep.

One last note. If you didn't know, Patrick is my middle name. The story I told at the beginning of the chapter is about myself. It's a true story about a time I struggled with sleep. After that first horrendous presentation and having taken the advice of my mum, I developed the Mind Wipe technique and of course tested it and used it on myself first. Developing good sleep habits and being properly prepared for my TED talk meant that that talk remained in the top 20 TED talks of all time for almost 20 years and at the time of writing has amassed over 18.5 million views. That one performance changed my life. Sleep is indeed magical.

MIND WIPE: FOUR STEPS TO REMEMBER

1. Imagine that you are in a room by yourself that has nothing else in it except four white wipeable walls, with the word ALERT written on each one inside a rectangle.
2. Using a tiny eraser, start to wipe the rectangle, followed by the word ALERT in real time, working backwards from the T.
3. When you've finished erasing the word from one board, wipe the word from the other three boards.
4. Taking a marker, write the word 'sleep' in lower case on the top left of the whiteboard, writing repeatedly until the board is full.

GALACTIC MIND WIPE: FOUR STEPS TO REMEMBER

1. Visualise your mind as the galaxy with thousands of stars, each symbolising a different worry, memory or thought.
2. Single out the stars shining most brightly – ten or so – and assign a specific worry or memory to each.
3. Visualise each of these stars transforming into shooting stars, streaking away and disappearing, until all the brightest stars have vanished.
4. Bathe in the tranquillity of your new mental gallery, free from intrusive, negative thoughts.

Well done! You've now read the second section, Psychological. I'm excited to lead you into the third section of the book, the Hypnomagical section, the final section, where you will learn to deploy some amazing techniques that will allow you to get restful, wonderful sleep.

PART 3: HYPNOMAGICAL

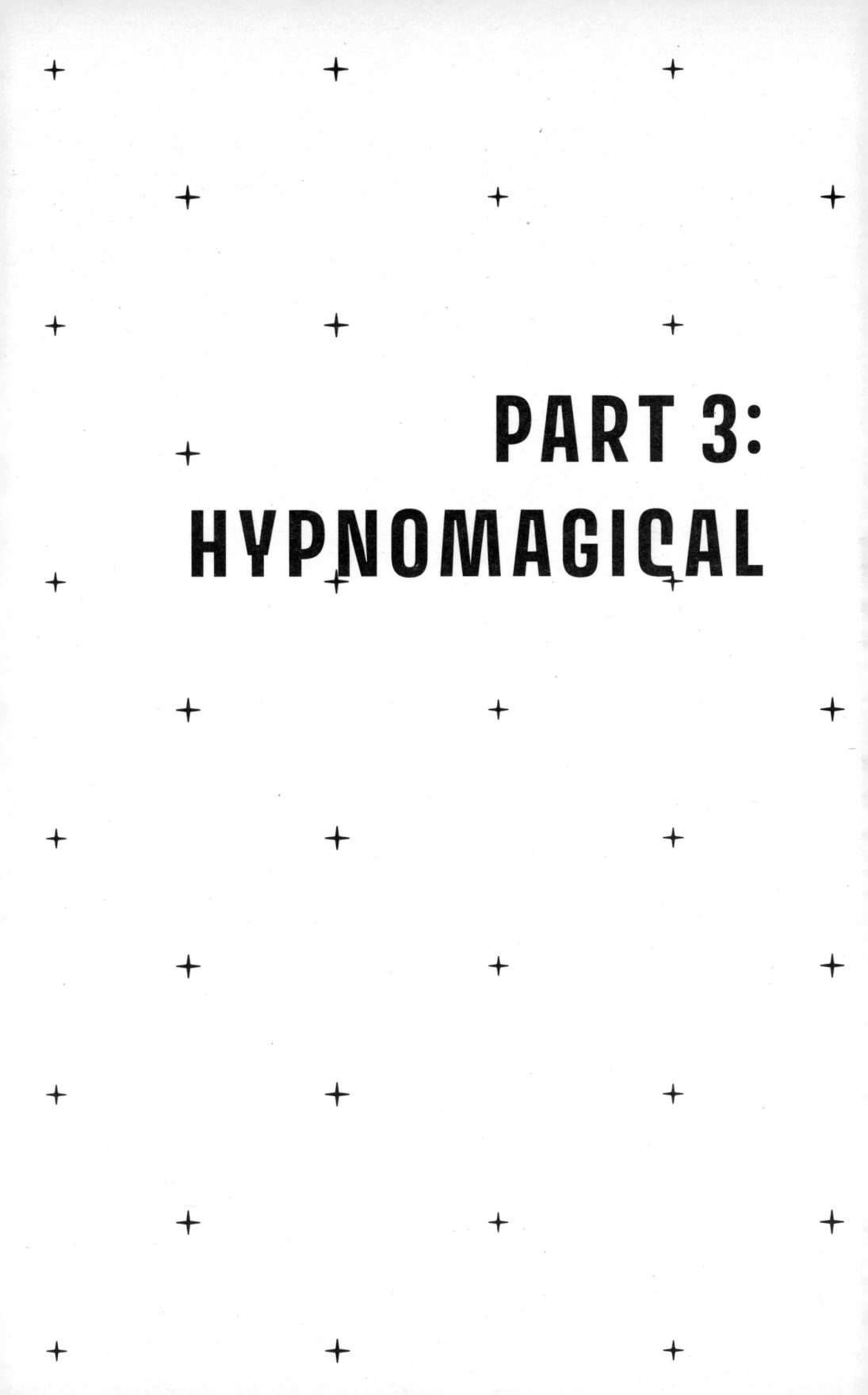

8

THE DREAMBOUND DESCENT

Welcome to the hypnomagical part of the book. In this section, I'm going to explain how you can hack your subconscious mind using a variety of unique hypnomagical techniques to relax you into a great sleep.

WHAT DOES HYPNOMAGICAL MEAN?

Working with the subconscious mind is at the core of everything that I do. Sure, people know the term 'subconscious' and they'll pepper their conversation with it, but very few people have even a basic understanding of the subconscious, let alone comprehend how they can access it to create permanent and sustainable change.

Simply put, your subconscious mind is where your memories, beliefs, urges, emotions and thoughts are all housed. It regulates your autonomic nervous system, which in turn regulates your heart rate (on average your heart beats 60–100 times per minute), your blood flow (through approximately 65,000 miles of blood vessels in your body), and your breathing (on average 12–20 breaths a minute). It also houses your fears and anxieties and, on a positive note, it is where your imagination lies.

Sometimes called the 'unconscious' mind, neuroscientists estimate that the subconscious mind is responsible for approximately 95 per cent of our brain processing. Read that again and let it sink in. There is a consensus in the neuroscience community that a very large percentage of our behaviours are driven by our subconscious mind rather than our conscious mind. And if you think about it for a moment, when you are asleep your subconscious mind is not only keeping you alive, it is also providing you with dreams – or nightmares. The good news is you can learn to hack your subconscious mind using what I call hypnomagical techniques.

There are six Hypnomagical Sleep Hacks over the next three chapters.

Remember, you're choosing one technique from Sleep Hacks 16–21 to combine with one Physical Sleep Hack and one Psychological Sleep Hack.

When I worked as a cosmetic scientist I would cycle 12.5km from Sandyford to Bray every day. There were many days when, as I clocked in, I barely remembered the cycle and as my finger hit the security keypad I would think to myself, 'Wow, I can't remember the past 45 minutes.' I had done the route so many times the repetitions had ingrained the action of cycling to work into my subconscious mind.

When was the last time you thought about your kidneys working? When was the last time you thought about brushing your teeth? Or driving the car? Or using the bathroom? All these processes happen subconsciously and of the 50,000–70,000 thoughts you have per day only a fraction are conscious. So you must learn how to quieten the subconscious mind and program it for deep, restorative sleep.

I call this **hypnomagical** thinking. The reason I've labelled the following techniques 'hypnomagical' is (a) because the techniques were born out of my background as a hypnotist, and (b) if done correctly they can achieve magical results.

The techniques involve a fusion of hypnotic principles, breathwork and magical thinking designed to guide your mind into a tranquil state, which will enable you to get the rest you desire. These techniques will serve as a bridge between alertness and the deep delta brainwave state necessary for restful slumber.

The subconscious is doing an awful lot of work underneath the surface. We are hit with so much information all the time (it's estimated that our brain processes somewhere close to 11 million pieces of information per second), and it's our subconscious that decides what parts to pass on to the conscious mind. When you learn something – driving, walking, operating your smartphone, how to button your coat – it becomes automatic and you don't have to think about it any more, and that's thanks to your subconscious mind. The subconscious has also been described as habitual. It has programs or habits ingrained within which happen automatically without us thinking about them, so once we start repeatedly doing an activity, it becomes part of our routine.

You can see where I'm going with this. Tap into your subconscious and you can change the way you feel and act, and this also applies to sleep.

Before I lead you into the first of my subconscious relaxation techniques for sleep, I'd like you to try some breathwork that will really help. This can also be used at times when you feel anxious and want to control your breathing and it's a very effective technique for settling your limbic system (the area in our brain associated with emotions and behaviour) and autonomic nervous system (the part that regulates involuntary processes like breathing and digestion). If you are combining breathwork with my hypno-magical techniques, you will really begin to harness the power of your subconscious mind and learn how to self-hypnotise yourself to sleep.

According to numerous studies, it is recommended that you breathe through your nose when preparing for and trying to get to sleep. There are several compelling reasons why it's the best way to breathe for getting some decent shut-eye.

First, if you're a snorer, your sleeping companion will really appreciate this. Engaging in nasal breathing can help reduce snoring by diminishing the tendency to breathe through the mouth, which in turns helps prevent you from sounding like a chainsaw buzzing as you wheeze the night away. This is because, when you breathe through your mouth, your soft palate, your tongue and your neck muscles all relax and this leads to you potentially reverberating with each breath.

If you breathe through your nose when you're sleeping, you're also less likely to wake up the next day with the dreaded 'morning breath' – this is most definitely another plus.

Your nose is also your safeguard against viruses, allergens and bacteria. When you breathe through the mouth, the air you're inhaling is unfiltered, whereas your nose collects all these potential pollutants and destroys them with enzymes before they can enter your body and make you sick.

Another reason to stop mouth breathing at night is that nasal breathing optimises your oxygen intake and allows your body to take in the correct amount of oxygen that your body needs.

Nasal breathing is also great for your oral health. If you're using your mouth to breathe, it means your gums and tongue become dried out. This leads to excess acids in the mouth, which can hasten tooth decay.

Last, but by no means least, breathing through the nose reduces the chances of you developing sleep apnoea. This is a sleep disorder in which your breathing stops and starts while you slumber. This obviously disrupts your sleep, and negatively impacts your quality of life. Even more alarmingly, sleep apnoea is linked to a range of health problems, including heart disease and stroke. This is not a road anybody wants to go down.

So if you're a night-time mouth breather, how do you stop it?

People often breathe through their mouth because their nasal passage is blocked. This can be remedied by using a neti pot or a saline spray to open up your nasal airways, or trying a nasal strip designed to help with decongestion. You could also try a different pillow and experiment with different heights, or materials, to allow you to prop your head up more in bed. Also, sleeping on your back is more likely to encourage you to breathe through your mouth, so sleep on your side instead.

If you consciously breathe through your nose whilst exercising or going for a walk you can begin to rewire your brain to become more of a nasal breather.

You may have also come across mouth taping. It's a popular trend on TikTok, and is championed by many well-known people, including renowned Stanford University neuroscientist Professor Andrew Huberman. Mouth taping involves taping your mouth before going to sleep so that you will then breathe through your nose. Mouth taping fans cite a whole host of benefits including better sleep and a reduction in bad breath. Hands up, I tried it once and found it wasn't for me; and a lot of the reported benefits are anecdotal. Actually, the night I tried it I whipped off the tape in the middle of the night and threw it on my nightstand. It fluttered gracefully from there onto the floor and I went back into a nice deep sleep. The next morning, the tape had glued itself to our brand new bedroom carpet, so you can imagine the interesting words my wife, Mairead, had for me when she noticed! It took a razor blade and an hour of patience to fix. But I digress. There have only been a couple of small scientific studies into the claim. One study of mild sleep apnoea found that among patients who had their lips taped shut, their snoring improved and the severity of their mild sleep apnoea declined.[30]

If you want to try mouth taping, speak to your GP first because there are no medically recognised guidelines on how to do it. And if you do, make sure that you use a porous tape designed for use on human skin. Otherwise, you run the risk of irritating your lips and the skin around your mouth; and if you have a beard, ripping it off can hurt like hell. Also, it's important to note that people who have anxiety shouldn't try mouth taping, because the idea of having their mouth taped shut might increase their feelings of anxiety.

Now it's time to learn how you can harness the mightiness of breathwork.

TRY THIS: UNLOCK THE POWER OF BREATH FOR DEEPER SLEEP

The foundation – deep breathing for tranquillity
Start by lying down and placing your hands on your belly. Begin with a deep breath in through your nose, filling your belly first and then your chest, for a count of four. Hold that breath for just a moment, allowing your lungs to fully expand. Now, exhale slowly through your mouth for a count of four. Repeat this calming pattern until you feel a sense of peace washing over you. Focus on the temperature of the air and how it feels as it oxygenates your body.

Tailor your breath to your needs
Customise your breathwork by adjusting the inhale–exhale ratio. Inhale for a count of four and exhale for a count of ten for a deeper sense of relaxation. Experiment with different patterns to find the rhythm that resonates best with your body. There is no right or wrong way to use breathwork. The important thing is the intention. The intention to focus on the breath and the relaxation it brings. We all vibrate at different frequencies so experimentation is the key to finding what rhythm works for you.

Mindful focus – engage the diaphragm, nose and mouth

Redirect your attention to your diaphragm, the muscle just below your ribcage that is responsible for deep breaths. Feel it expand as you inhale and release as you exhale. Welcome the effects of nasal breathing, allowing the air to be filtered and humidified. Integrate the power of both the nose and mouth in your breathwork, maximising the intake of oxygen and the focus of the exhale through the mouth.

Establish a routine for sustainable sleep

Incorporate this breathwork into your nightly routine in preparation for self-hypnosis. As you consistently practise, it will become a sign and a signal to your body that it's time to unwind and prepare for rest. Over time, this routine will become a powerful sleep-inducing habit.

Repeat the process until you are fully comfortable, calm and relaxed.

Be sure to embrace this journey, experiment with the techniques, and witness the positive impact on your sleep quality and overall wellbeing.

The idea behind breathwork is that it is bringing oxygen into your body, helping to alleviate stress, which in turn makes you feel more balanced. While it's very on-trend right now, it actually dates back thousands of years, with its roots lying in yoga practices.

It has lots of significant potential health benefits. For example, breathwork has been shown to alkalise your blood pH (an acidic blood pH accelerates ageing), it has an anti-inflammatory effect, and it is a mood elevator. This is because when you breathe deeply and slowly, your brain tells your body that everything is okay, and that it's safe to relax. This can help balance your blood pressure, allows you more time in deep sleep and improves your respiratory function.

THE MAGICAL WORLD OF DREAMS

A recent investigation conducted by Aberystwyth University's psychology department, exploring magicians worldwide, suggests that people involved in the field of illusion and magic may experience fewer mental health challenges compared to both other creative professionals and the general population.[31]

The study analysed psychopathological traits in nearly 200 magicians, contrasting the findings with data from various artistic groups and the overall population. The research determined that magicians exhibited notably lower scores in comparison to other creative individuals and the general public. Despite their profession revolving around creating illusions and delving into the mysterious, magicians were found to be less susceptible to unusual phenomena like hallucinations or cognitive disorganisation.

I believe part of the reason magicians are less susceptible to psychopathological disorders is our ability to control our subconscious thoughts and induce creativity and magical thinking.

I have used the following technique, Dreambound Descent, for many years to promote my own creativity and problem-solving abilities and I find it an amazing way to completely free my mind in order to spark innovative perspectives.

Magicians are known as dreamers. But what if I told you that you can program your dreams? Not only that, you can then use your dreams to approach everyday challenges with a heightened sense of creativity and focus. And as a result you will potentially be less prone to mental illness.

Let's take a deep dive into the magical world of dreams – a terrain where the mind is capable of crazy, weird, wacky and wondrous dreams and literally anything is possible. Dreams aren't just a nightly Netflix binge for your brain; they're a treasure trove of untapped potential. It's time now to tap into that untapped potential and unlock the 95 per cent of your brain that is normally outside your awareness. We're going to explore how dreams can be your secret weapon for supercharged creativity and increased problem-solving abilities.

CREATIVITY AND DREAMING

Dreams aren't just the mind's late-night improv show; they're a breeding ground for creativity that can blow your conscious, waking thoughts out of the water. Think of them as your brain's after-hours party where the rules of reality get tossed out of the window. Dreams have an extraordinary ability to pull ideas out of thin air, making the impossible seem downright doable.

STRESS ALLEVIATION THROUGH DREAM THERAPY

Now let's talk about dreams as your personal therapist. Dreams aren't just bizarre video reels or cartoons playing in your head; they're also a system for processing your emotions. Stress, fears and anxiety get a symbolic, metaphorical makeover in dreamland. It's your brain's way of saying, 'Let's sort this mess out, shall we?' Imagine Dreambound Descent as a guided tour of your subconscious, where you can not only sort out the mess, but also actively influence the outcome of your dreams before they even begin!

INDUCING LUCID DREAMS: YOUR TICKET TO DREAM EXPLORATION

Let's crank it up a notch with some lucid dreaming action. It's time to become the Steven Spielberg of your own blockbuster dream. My favourite quote of all time is from Spielberg: 'I don't just dream at night. I dream all day. I dream for a living.' It doesn't matter what job or role you are in; you have an imagination that can fuel your dreams. And whatever your circumstances you can choose whether or not to think like Spielberg. That's where lucid dreaming kicks in. It's like having a TV remote control for your brain, and you're the batteries that control the remote.

TRY THIS: TRIGGER A LUCID DREAM Three times during the day, close your eyes, ignite your imagination and visualise 60-second dreams. If you find it difficult to visualise, simply imagine you can visualise! Daydream of anything at all. Climbing that mountain. Winning that competition. Retiring to Hawaii. Whatever. Hold that thought for the full 60 seconds and really feel yourself experiencing how wonderful it is, and how good achieving this goal will make you feel. Do this regularly, and your brain will start pulling the same mind games in your dreams, triggering that sweet lucidity.

On average, people experience multiple dreams during a single night's sleep. The exact number can vary, but most individuals have several dreams, typically between four and six, every night. Dreams obviously vary in length, but they generally last between five and 20 minutes. However, the perception of time in dreams is distorted and is much different from real life.

Most vivid dreaming occurs during REM (rapid eye movement) sleep, which is one of the stages of the natural sleep cycle. REM sleep usually occurs multiple times throughout the night, and the length of each REM period increases with each cycle.

Lucid dreaming is a phenomenon where the dreamer becomes aware that they are dreaming and may have some degree of control over their dream. It's a skill that you can cultivate over time with Dreambound Descent.

Dreams may also play a role in memory consolidation. Some research suggests that dreaming helps to process and consolidate memories, allowing the brain to sift through and organise information gathered during waking hours.

But dreams are still something of a mystery to scientists.

Brain activity during REM is closest to our brain activity when we are awake, but the scientific community isn't 100 per cent sure what REM sleep's function is, and what the function of dreaming is. Certainly, it's thought to be important for brain development. Newborns spend most of their early lives in REM sleep, and the amount of REM sleep gets less and less, plateauing in early adulthood. It stays the same throughout adulthood, until later in life when REM sleep levels reduce and sleep can become more fragmented. REM sleep is also thought to facilitate learning. One theory is that the brain sorts and filters connections made during the day, keeping the connections that are useful and getting rid of the ones we don't need.

By embracing the power of dreams and throwing in some

brain-hacking techniques, you're not just catching some zzzs; you're unleashing the full potential of your mind.

Although most of the hacks in this book are used to enter into a calm and soothing sleep, remember that Dreambound Descent can be used for hacking into the mind's hidden subconscious powers and can be used to create a blueprint for your goals and dreams. The emphasis here is on pushing boundaries and being open-minded, thinking beyond your limitations, and tackling grand challenges with creative, unconventional solutions in the freedom of deep sleep. It involves setting seemingly impossible goals that inspire and drive progress, even if the path to achieving them is uncertain or challenging.

In August 2020, I decided to run an experiment using Dreambound Descent. My only focus was on writing my new live show. I had no material, ideas or scripts written. The only word was the title – *Insanity*. I would focus on that word every night as I entered into sleep using Dreambound Descent. After 16 dreamless nights something magical occurred. I dreamt that the end of the show was a reveal to a trick with the audience raving to Mark McCabe's song 'Maniac' and imagining they were the actress Meg Ryan. I had no idea what this meant but I scribbled it into my creativity journal first thing the next morning. Five nights later I had another dream – the audience was imagining they were in Germany for a late-night rave. After another four nights, in my dream I realised that Meg Ryan was a symbol for something. Without using technology, can you guess what Meg Ryan is an anagram of? This was an amazing revelation. The hairs are standing up on the backs of my arms as I remember this. The end of the *Insanity* show became exactly that: a full-on rave where the audience themselves became the end of the show. A mind-reading show that ended with a rave! The energy was electric and the whole ending came from my dreams! But I am not alone: throughout history, many notable people have been inspired by their dreams.

Have you heard of Elias Howe? He was born in Massachusetts in the US in 1819. It was a time when everything had to be sewn by hand. He worked in a shop, and then one night he had the most amazing dream. In the dream, he was surrounded by cannibals who wanted to eat him and were waving spears at him. When he woke up, he recalled that the spears had holes in the shaft that moved up and down. This led to his invention of the sewing machine, and the innovative lock stitch, which uses a needle with a thread that goes up and down, entwining in a hole in the fabric. It's fair to say that this invention revolutionised sewing and made Elias Howe a very rich man. Weirdly, there's a link between Elias and the next big name who found inspiration in their dreams. At the end of the Beatles' 1965 film *Help*, there is a credit that reads, 'This film is respectfully dedicated to the memory of Mr. Elias Howe, who, in 1846, invented the sewing machine.' Why have a dedication to Elias? Nobody is sure. But perhaps it's linked to Paul McCartney's experience of lucid dreaming. In 1963, the melody for 'Yesterday', one of the best songs ever written, came to him in a dream. He awoke and rushed to the piano to work out the chords. 'I just fell out of bed, found out what key I had dreamed it in … and I played it,' he recalled later.

Author Mary Shelley came up with *Frankenstein* following a dream, and Robert Louis Stevenson similarly found inspiration for *Dr Jekyll and Mr Hyde* from his dreams.

When you look at the world of science, you'll find a whole heap of lucid dreamers whose nocturnal imaginings turned out to be life-changing. August Kekulé, a nineteenth-century German organic chemist, was the first to visualise the ring structure of benzene, a discovery that enabled it to be developed in laboratories; it's an important chemical in many production processes. The idea came to him during a period of lucid dreaming, when he saw a snake eating its own tail.

Albert Einstein said that he discovered the theory of relativity in a dream. Serbian-American futurist and inventor Nikola Tesla, who is best known for his contributions to the electricity system and who is widely regarded as a genius, used lucid dreaming to conduct experiments without having to actually physically do them, which then helped him identify problems in his ideas.

Dmitri Mendeleev came up with the final form of the periodic table of elements while dreaming, while Otto Loewi scooped the Nobel Prize in medicine after discovering the role of a particular neurotransmitter, again while he was asleep.

I recently used Dreambound Descent for writing my current live show, *Mind Games*. I simply sketched out a brain with the words Mind Games written inside the brain. I stared at it every night for 60 seconds, followed by breathwork and Dreambound Descent. Unlike my *Insanity* show, the ideas came fast and thick straight away on night one. I think this is because of the dozens and dozens of times I have practised the technique. I envisaged myself reading the whole audience's minds under scientific test conditions, and saw myself selling out the Bord Gáis Energy Theatre. Over several subsequent nights, the whole script came to me too. I'm delighted to say I performed *Mind Games* recently to a sold-out audience in the Bord Gáis with everyone in attendance having their mind read. Dreams really do come true!

You see, our subconscious mind, when free from waking activity, has the ability during sleep to seek novel connections and offer solutions to problems.

TRY THIS: USE YOUR DREAMS TO PROBLEM-SOLVE
> Place a dream journal next to your bed.
> In your dream journal write down a problem you want to solve or a subject you want to dream about, in fewer than ten words.
> Convert that problem or subject into a simple doodle. Your mind processes images 60,000 times faster than text, so converting your target into a picture is key (that's why I drew a brain with the words Mind Games in the centre for developing my current theatre show).
> Set your intention before you go to sleep that you will remember your dreams.
> Enter into the Dreambound Descent process described below with an open mind.
> Scribble down your nocturnal adventures as soon as you wake up.

It's like hacking into your brain's secret stash of inspiration. Trust the process and let your subconscious work its magic. Dreams aren't just passive entertainment; they're the backstage pass to your brain's personal magic show.

Now you're ready to try this, one of my go-to techniques to take control of the subconscious mind, induce amazing lucid dreams and relax into a deep creative sleep. It's a visionary and unusual approach to hacking your subconscious creative landscape and utilising the stress-busting power of dreams.

SLEEP HACK 16
DREAMBOUND DESCENT

An audio recording where I guide you through this visualisation can be accessed on my website www.keithbarry.com/sleephacks with the password SLEEPHACKS24.

In this technique, you're going to visualise your own personal sleep stairs. And at the end of that sleep stairs is the most serene, beautiful sleep space you could ever possibly imagine.

- › Begin by lying down and closing your eyes. You are now going to practise your deep breathing. Take a long, calming deep breath in through your nose, filling your lungs with fresh, soothing, calming oxygen, and exhale through your mouth, releasing any lingering tension from your body or mind. Do this five times.
- › Now visualise a beautiful staircase. It is the most majestic staircase you have ever seen, and it is a deep and beautiful shade of purple.
- › You are standing at the top of this purple staircase. And as you look down, you notice that your feet are bare. Underneath your bare feet is the most luxurious, soft, cushiony, purple carpet that you have ever seen. Visualise the staircase again in your mind's eye. Now, this is no ordinary staircase. It is

your sleep stairs, and it has been designed by the architect of your own mind's eye to lead you gently and naturally into a state of restful sleep.

- Now, this staircase is dimly lit with soft, glowing lights that cast a gentle soothing glow on each step. This light is pale blue in colour, casting a shadow on every step of your purple stairs. Visualise these steps in your mind's eye. Decide yourself if they are wide and sturdy or if they're narrow and fragile.
- Use your own imagination to decide how wide the handrail is. Now notice how smooth the handrail is. In your mind, see if you notice any flaws in the handrail, but all the time observing how beautiful this scene is, how beautiful this staircase it, and how calming it already feels to just visualise this staircase.
- In a moment, in your mind you're going to start descending the stairs. You are aware with every step you take down those stairs that your conscious mind, your subconscious mind and your super-subconscious mind will relax deeper and deeper towards that wonderful night's sleep that you so truly desire.
- You now notice how many steps there are on this staircase. You observe that there are 50 steps in total, and that it's a spiral staircase. As you gaze at the staircase, right down to the bottom, you can see that in the very centre there's a library. It's huge and filled with ancient books containing the collective dreams of humanity.
- You know that you must take 50 steps down the purple staircase so that you can begin to explore those intriguing books. Beginning at 50, as you descend, all the concerns and

anxieties of the day just dissipate and disappear. You find yourself immediately becoming more relaxed. With every step you take down that stairs you find your mind, body and soul becoming more relaxed. For the first 10 steps down the stairs, repeat the mantra 'I am calm, relaxed and ready to dream.' You first descend to step 49. This is a peaceful step that guides you into a feeling of deep relaxation.

> Now on to step 48, a peaceful step that deepens your relaxation. Always remember to breathe in through your nose and out through your mouth. Remind yourself to be in the present moment. Yesterday is gone. Tomorrow is a new day. Right here, right now, in this moment, all that matters is your intention to sleep and induce interesting and intriguing dreams.

> You now move down to step 47. Notice now how your breathing is beginning to settle. That's a signal to your mind, your body and your soul to relax your autonomic nervous system, which is your heart rate, your blood pressure, your digestive system. They all begin to settle down and work in unison to help you relax even more.

> Descending down the steps, as you hit step 46, and for all the other steps, right down to the last step where the library of your imagination awaits you, I want to you to say three times silently to yourself:
I feel relaxed, drowsy and sleepy
I feel relaxed, drowsy and sleepy
I feel relaxed, drowsy and sleepy.

- Repeat this at every step and continue to go down the staircase. You may find yourself drifting into a deep, restful slumber at step 39 or 21 and if that happens that's perfectly fine.

> If you manage to make your way all the way down the 50 steps to the last step, visualise yourself entering the library of your mind. Take a moment to explore your library and take note of any information you discover in the pages of the books you find. You notice how quiet, peaceful and calm it is in that library. You are entering a deep and restful night's sleep. Then, something strange happens. In your sleep, in the library, you begin to dream. Your dream is déjà vu, because you begin again at step 50 and move down to step 49. You're beginning the process all over again, in your dream. Once again, you're descending, in your dream, down the stairs. This is like an infinity loop dream and it continues to happen again and again and again in your mind.

If you can commit to doing this, you cannot help but fall asleep and have the most profound and amazing journey into an abyss of dreams.

Did you guess what Meg Ryan is an anagram of? Germany! At the end of my *Insanity* theatre show the audience danced and raved as Meg Ryan in a nightclub in Germany. (It was one of those 'you had to be there' moments.)

DREAMBOUND DESCENT: FIVE STEPS TO REMEMBER

> Visualise yourself at the top of a purple spiral staircase.
> Practise your deep breathing before going down, a step at a time.
> On the third step, and for every step afterwards, repeat the mantra 'I am relaxed, drowsy and sleepy' three times.

> Continue on down for 50 steps until you climb into a comfortable bed.
> If you are still awake at this point, imagine you are dreaming that you are at the top of the stairs again, and repeat the process.

Remember, if this Hypnomagical Sleep Hack doesn't appeal to you or doesn't work for you, there are five other Hypnomagical techniques to try in the following chapters.

9

THE SLEEPSCAPE GARDEN

In the hustle and bustle of modern life, it seems to me that we have lost the ability to connect with nature. In the previous chapters in this book we have explored innovative, modern, technological and holistic approaches to achieving a rejuvenating night's sleep. But what if it was even simpler than you could have possibly imagined?

In this, the second chapter in the Hypnomagical section, I'm introducing you to a unique idea that I developed and refined recently: the concept of the Sleepscape Garden, a mental sanctuary where you can cultivate specific plants, flowers and trees associated with relaxation and peace. Even if you think you don't have green fingers and this is not for you, please don't skip this chapter. It may well be the solution you are looking for.

Once again, this Sleep Hack is one of the six hacks you can choose from in this section, to be combined with one from the Physical section and one from Psychological. But first …

MEET KEN

A client of mine, Ken, aged 75, woke up on Wednesday 22 February 2023 struggling to speak. He put it down to the excess lemon he had had on his pancakes the previous day, Pancake Tuesday. He waited a few days before going to a doctor, but after the doctor's visit his voice deteriorated even more. Over the course of a few weeks and after many scopes, ultrasounds and X-rays the diagnosis came out of the blue. He was diagnosed with stage 4 lung cancer. For a man who never smoked this truly came as a shock. The tumours were not only in his lungs but also in his back and various lymph nodes. By December 2023, his body had been blasted with two doses of radiation, six bouts of intense chemotherapy plus two doses of less intense chemotherapy. Initially, the intense chemotherapy seemed to do the trick – the tumours had shrunk and he was feeling better overall. He was then due to stay on the less intense maintenance chemo for life in an attempt to stop the cancer from spreading even further. However, after just two sessions of the maintenance chemotherapy he got the call to go to hospital and to bring someone with him. His wife and son accompanied Ken and knew they were most likely facing bad news. Sure enough, the oncologist explained that the cancer had spread further and he quickly needed different treatment. The new treatment involved a trial drug, which the doctors weren't sure if they could get, as Ken needed to be tested for his eligibility for the trial.

Throughout all of this his sleep suffered. He was uncomfortable in bed most nights with pain in his left lung, and the nights when he had little or no pain the 'what if' thoughts kept him awake most nights: What if I don't get the trial drug? What if it spreads to my back and I end up in a wheelchair? What if I end up in a hospice? What if I can't see my grandkids grow up?

I worked with Ken on improving his sleep using a variety of techniques from this book, with mixed results. He successfully used the Magic of the Black Balloon and Mind Wipe techniques and also, under his doctor's supervision, added some natural foods to his diet, such as goji berries, sardines and almonds, to help increase his melatonin levels in order to aid his sleep. The change in diet worked sporadically but not every night. The good news was that Ken is a determined man and he was willing to explore every technique until he found the one that worked for him. The technique that did work for him is the Sleepscape Garden visualisation that follows. He uses it every single night now to attain a deep six hours' unbroken sleep. Every single night! Although, as you know, seven hours is optimal, for Ken at this stage, six hours is almost magical.

THE (REALLY) GREAT OUTDOORS

We'll get back to Ken in a while, but for now here's something about me that few people know. I love gardening! Most people think I'm from Dublin, as my accent is mostly Dublin with a hint of Galway, but I am proud to say I'm a Waterford man through and through. I was born and bred in Williamstown, which back in 1976 was a narrow, country road with a row of houses and surrounded by fields. I'm actually a culchie. My grandparents on my mother's side, Lizzie and Johnny, used to live next door to us. Johnny (Gaga) was a gardener/landscaper by trade and grew his own fruit and vegetables all year round on the half acre or so of land surrounding their house.

I would help him with the plot, from which we would process fresh, homegrown produce for our meals. Whether it was planting seeds, nurturing newly sprouted plants, or tending to the flourishing garden beds, the shared effort brought us closer together. As the seasons unfolded, we reaped the rewards of our hard work, harvesting an abundance of organic vegetables and fruits. As I look back on those youthful days, I can tell you one thing for certain: I slept soundly every single night in my prepubescent years. Recently I began to wonder how and why I slept so deeply.

I'm guessing it's because of a number of factors. In my tweens (aged 10–13 for those of you who don't know!) I had very few worries. I was exercising daily – either playing soccer or out and about exploring on my BMX bicycle. I obviously wasn't drinking alcohol, I read a lot and I was also already good at understanding the power of visualisation. But I also now believe part of the reason I slept so soundly was my deep connection with nature. If I wasn't gardening with Gaga (which was almost every day) I was outside doing something else, like climbing trees, stealing apples from orchards, trying to catch frogs; or, at the weekend, I was picking cockles, mushrooms or periwinkles or fishing with my dad – all outside in nature, no matter what the weather was like.

And now, as an adult, I make a point of going into my small back garden every single day, whatever the weather. Whether it's to plant new bulbs for spring, ground myself, cut the grass, or to get into my ice bath, I make it part of my ritual to get into the garden daily, even for just a few minutes. I love springtime the most because that's when I can plant new vegetables such as carrots, peas, potatoes, etc. Even if you don't have a garden, or you think gardening is just not for you, please do read on, because I have a gardening technique for you to use that only requires your mind.

WHY GARDENING IS SO GOOD

We are so disconnected with nature now it's actually frightening. Although a quick walk in nature at the weekend is beneficial, I would argue it's simply not enough to aid our sleep.

Let's delve into the reasons we should all be gardening, its potential sleep benefits, and how, if you have no garden or no interest in the physical activity of gardening, you can still create your own mental sleep garden.

Gardening, in its physical form, has been a cherished activity across cultures and centuries. The earliest sign of gardening in Ireland dates back to Neolithic times, around 6,000 years ago. The oldest continuously cultivated garden in Ireland is most likely the Upper Garden in Lismore Castle, County Waterford, which dates back to around 1605.

Whether it's a small community plot, a tiny corner garden, herbs in a window box or a potted plant in the corner of a room, people worldwide find peace and tranquillity in nurturing living things. Bringing plants to life and seeing them flourish and grow has an inherent therapeutic quality, connecting people to the wonders of nature and reducing their cortisol levels. Gardening should have a universal appeal, and to say 'it doesn't interest me' or 'I don't have green fingers' just further highlights the need to think deeply about this subject and the impact it can have on overall wellbeing and, indeed, your sleep. In order to aid our sleep patterns, we need to deeply reconnect with nature to counteract the amount of time we are spending mindlessly scrolling on devices. Studies have consistently shown that exposure to nature, even just imagining being in nature, can reduce stress, lower cortisol levels, and improve overall wellbeing, both psychologically and physiologically, which as a result will yield deeper and better-quality sleep.

For example, a study in the Netherlands indicated that a 10 per cent increase in exposure to green space translated into an improvement to health equivalent to being five years younger.[32] Studies in Japan and Canada have also found similar benefits. In children and young people, green spaces have been linked with reduced levels of obesity in children in America and the proportion of green spaces is linked to self-reported improved levels of mental health.

A very interesting 2016 report from the UK outlined the myriad of benefits that gardening brings, ranging from reduced depression and anxiety to improved social functioning.[33] Of course, it can be a calorie-intense activity too, and half an hour of gardening will burn the same amount of calories as half an hour playing badminton or volleyball!

A recent study discovered that for people who gardened daily, compared to someone who didn't garden at all, their wellbeing scores were higher.[34]

Stop for a moment and give some deep, meaningful thought to those results. In basic terms, people who garden are almost twice as likely to have better mental health than those who don't. I don't know about you but I'd much rather be gardening than popping an antidepressant pill or a sleeping tablet – and again I'm going to share with you how you can do this without getting your hands dirty if you don't fancy going into the garden or don't have access to one.

TRY THIS: CREATE A BIOPHILIC BEDROOM Create a calm environment in your bedroom by adding elements of nature into the design. Consider things like shells from a beach, artwork made from twigs, sand art, an indoor plant or any nature-inspired paintings. These will help foster a connection with the natural world, which may work wonders for your sleep.

TRY THIS: GREEN UP YOUR BEDROOM As well as looking beautiful, indoor plants have a lots of benefits. They've been shown to alleviate stress levels and if they're gently fragranced, they can also contribute to a feeling of calm. Lavender, jasmine, peace lilies and gardenia are all plants associated with sleep that you can keep in your bedroom, as well as spider plants (bonus: it's difficult to kill these, even if you're a neglectful plant parent) and aloe vera.

THE ART OF SHINRIN-YOKU

Let's take a trip to Japan. It's the country where the mindfulness practice shinrin-yoku originated. Shinrin-yoku, also known as forest bathing, arose in the 1980s as a response to tech burnout and also to encourage Japanese people to become reacquainted with their forests and nature in general. It's a very simple thing to do. It means being calm and quiet among the trees, observing the nature around you, and breathing deeply as you immerse yourself in the forest's atmosphere.

It is a deeply relaxing, sensory experience, one where you're not rushing, not thinking about your to-do lists, but smelling, feeling and absorbing the restorative effects of nature. Dr Qing Li writes in his book *Shinrin-Yoku: The Art and Science of Forest Bathing*:

Make sure you have left your phone and camera behind. You are going to be walking aimlessly and slowly. You don't need any devices. Let your body be your guide. Listen to where it wants to take you. Follow your nose. And take your time. It doesn't matter if you don't get anywhere. You are not going anywhere. You are savouring the sounds, smells and sights of nature and letting the forest in.

You can certainly do your own, unstructured forest bathing. But if you think you might need some guidance, you can check the Tree Council of Ireland's website (www.treecouncil.ie) for a list of forest bathing guides who each offer different kinds of experiences. These range from forest bath songs (singing in the forest) to nature connection workshops.

Although Japan coined the term for this practice, it has been known for a long time, by many cultures, that connecting with nature has many benefits. But what exactly does that have to do with sleep? A lot, actually. A study of middle-aged men investigated the effects of forest bathing on serotonin levels, depressive symptoms and subjective sleep quality.[35] It found that forest bathing significantly increased serotonin levels and decreased the participants' fatigue score. Interestingly, it also led to a reduction in morning sleepiness.

Unless you're lucky enough to have some woods or a forest on your doorstep, if you do try forest bathing, it's probably going to be a weekend activity. Maybe the tree huggers are not crazy after all!

TRY THIS: GROUND YOURSELF If you have a garden, something that you could do every day is to spend 10 to 30 minutes walking barefoot outside, a practice that is also known as grounding, or earthing, where the human body reconnects with the Earth's electrical charge and healing energy. It's currently an under-researched area but some of the studies that have been done into grounding are promising and it is something I practise myself.

These studies have centred on how grounding relates to inflammation, heart disease, muscle damage, mood and sleep. One study from 2011 included four different experiments on grounding and its effect on the body.[36] The results showed that thyroid and glucose levels, electrolytes and immune response improved with grounding. One of the earliest published studies on grounding looked at its effect on sleep and circadian cortisol profiles. Twelve subjects who were in pain and had problems sleeping grounded for eight weeks. During this period, their night-time cortisol profiles became normal and most of the subjects reported that their sleep improved and their stress levels decreased.[37]

As I've said, more research needs to be done into grounding, but considering that we know it's beneficial to be outside, give grounding a shot and note how it makes you feel. You can walk barefoot on grass or earth, or sit up against a tree and feel the bark against your skin. It's probably not advisable to go barefoot in public parks, which might not be very sanitary, so if you don't have a garden or green space to walk in, you can always get a grounding mat. These can be picked up online and they're relatively inexpensive. These mats, which you plug into an electric socket, simulate the Earth's electrical current, and replace the direct contact with the earth that you'd get walking barefoot outside.

SLEEP HACK 17
SLEEPSCAPE GARDEN

An audio recording where I guide you through this visualisation can be accessed on my website www.keithbarry.com/sleephacks with the password SLEEPHACKS24.

The Sleepscape Garden takes our subconscious universal love of gardening (you might consciously disagree with that, but your subconscious mind knows it loves gardening – it's hardwired into your genetic code) and transforms it into a mental exercise with the aim of promoting better sleep. Creating your own Sleepscape Garden inside the inner recesses of your subconscious mind involves identifying specific plants or elements associated with relaxation, peace and tranquillity and mentally cultivating them into a personalised mental space. You will also imagine any unwanted or intrusive thoughts as weeds (which tend to keep us awake), which you will pull out and destroy, just as you would if you were tending to your own real garden.

> Lie down, close your eyes and begin to allow yourself to sink into a state of deep relaxation. Start with an awareness

of your body, and begin to picture yourself on the verge of sleep, with your body fully relaxed, your subconscious mind open to positive suggestions. This is the gateway to your Sleepscape Garden hypnotic ritual.

> Now, imagine a path with soft, luscious grass beneath your bare feet. As you walk slowly along this path you can see a beautiful garden in the distance. It begins to get closer and closer and more distinct with every careful step that you take.

> Imagine stepping into that vast, moonlit garden – this is your own personal Sleepscape Garden, a mental sanctuary designed exclusively by you for your wellbeing. You are an expert landscape gardener with all of the tools and techniques necessary to design your own perfectly manicured garden. Visualise this garden bathed in soft moonlight, the air filled with the calming scents of rose and lavender. Take a long, deep breath in and allow those soothing scents to permeate deep into your soul. There is a gentle breeze carrying the fragrance of blooming flowers and the earthy scent of the soil beneath your feet. As you step forward, become aware of the vibrant colours surrounding you – a kaleidoscope of greens, blues, purples and all the colours of the rainbow.

> In the heart of this mystical garden stands a majestic tree – your Tree of Serenity. Its branches stretch out gracefully, providing peace and comfort. This tree is the core of your peaceful existence. Picture it as a strong and solid symbol of all the positive thoughts, aspirations, targets and goals worth nurturing in your life. As you visualise, feel the roots

of this tree grounding you, connecting you to the essence of tranquillity.

- Around this tree, begin to plant seeds of serenity, each seed being a metaphor for a thought or emotion that brings you inner peace. One seed might represent gratitude, and the things you are thankful for in life. Another seed might represent forgiveness and the people in life you need to inwardly forgive. Others might represent compassion, positivity, self-love, and so on. Picture the seeds growing into vibrant plants and trees, transforming your inner world into a haven of calmness and peace. Take your time with this visualisation to grow as many flowers, trees and plants as you can think of, labelling each one with a positive thought or emotion as you do so.

- Begin to wander deeper into the garden, noticing an array of flowers in full bloom. Each flower represents even more positive aspects of your life. Picture them vividly – the vibrant red of passion, the soothing blue of calmness, the bright yellow of joy. The sleepiness of purple and the optimism of green. These flowers embody the positive thoughts that contribute to your overall wellbeing. Take a moment to appreciate their beauty and the positivity they bring to your mental landscape.

- As we progress, switch your focus back to your body. Feel the tension and any aches or pains you may have melting away. With each breath imagine you are feeding your inner garden with all the nutrients it needs, releasing that tension, allowing your whole body to relax, making way for the cultivation of calmness within.

- Now let's introduce a symphony of soothing sounds – the rustling leaves, the gentle breeze and the melodic language of the birds singing all around you in the moonlight. They weave together to create a harmonious melody, drowning out the hum of insomnia-induced concerns and guiding you deeper into relaxation. When you imagine these sounds really make an effort to turn up the volume in your mind to hear them loud and clear in your mind.
- Next, focus on the act of nurturing. Picture yourself tending to the Tree of Serenity, watering its roots with positivity and care. As you do so, acknowledge the positive thoughts and goals in your life, feeling a sense of gratitude for each one. Visualise them growing stronger, their branches reaching towards the sky, symbolising the fulfilment of your aspirations.
- In the process of cultivating your mental garden, it's essential to recognise and address any unwanted negativity. Imagine a small area where weeds have sprouted – these represent negative thoughts, doubts, or worries. With each breath, picture yourself pulling these weeds from the soil and destroying them in any way you want. Feel the weight lifting as you discard these unwanted intruders. This act symbolises your ability to let go of negativity and maintain your garden of tranquillity.
- As you explore your mental garden, consider expanding its boundaries. Visualise it growing beyond the immediate surroundings, spreading positivity and calmness throughout your entire being. Envisage this garden as a sanctuary you can retreat to at any moment, a place where the positive energy nurtures not only your sleep but every aspect of your life.

- Feel a connection with the natural rhythms of your garden. The gentle rustling of leaves in the breeze, the moonlight on your skin and the soothing sounds of a stream – these elements harmonise with the natural rhythms of your body. As you sync with these rhythms, imagine your internal clock aligning with the natural ebb and flow of day and night, resetting your circadian rhythm and contributing to a more restful and rejuvenating sleep.
- As you transition into the increasing darkness of night-time, notice your Sleepscape Garden quietening down and becoming still, signalling the approach of restful sleep. Imagine yourself lying on the soft grass gently descending into slumber, mirroring the subtle shift as the moonlight fades and the garden becomes dark.
- Now embrace the night. Trust in the power of your newly nurtured garden to keep your mind positive and safe as you sleep. Acknowledge that sleep is a natural, effortless yet important process. Picture your Sleepscape Garden shrouded in the velvety darkness of night, a place where restorative rest is not only possible but inevitable.
- As we come to the end of this visualisation, allow the imagery of your tranquil garden to linger. Stay in your Sleepscape Garden until you doze off in real life. The Tree of Serenity and the blooming flowers are now etched in your mind as powerful symbols of positivity and peace.

Remember, you have the power to cultivate this mental garden regularly. Use this visualisation whenever you need to centre yourself and promote restful sleep. If you find it hard to follow the flow of this visualisation, simply take a moment to sketch out your garden on a piece of paper or in your sleep journal. This may help you with the process.

While the primary focus is on improving sleep, the Sleepscape Garden concept extends beyond just sleep. The technique emphasises how the principles of the Sleepscape Garden can positively influence various aspects of daily life, from stress management to enhanced emotional intelligence.

KEN'S STORY, CONTINUED

To update you about Ken: he got the trial drug and at the time of writing he is doing well, considering the battering his mind and body have taken. He is sleeping soundly every single night by using the Sleepscape Garden technique, which is working wonders for his mood and outlook in the midst of a very difficult situation. In his Sleepscape Garden he digs the soil, which he rubs between his hands, and the smell reminds him of his childhood gardening with his father. He also sees a plump robin redbreast in his garden every night with the robin singing poetically as it flies gracefully from flower to flower and branch to branch. The robin reminds him again of his father and he takes comfort that his dad, Paddy, is at peace and looking out for him. As the saying goes, 'When robins appear, loved ones are near.'

A sceptic by nature, he certainly didn't believe that the technique would work for him, but he tried it anyway. I'm delighted it worked for him – in case you didn't guess already, Ken is my hero. My number one client. My best friend and mentor. He's my dad.

SLEEPSCAPE GARDEN: SEVEN STEPS TO REMEMBER

1. Relax your body fully and as you do so imagine a path of luscious grass under your bare feet, with a garden visible in the distance.
2. Walk slowly towards the moon-drenched garden, smelling the beautiful scent of the flowers and the earthy smell of the soil, while enjoying the gentle surroundings. Become aware of the vibrant colours surrounding you – a kaleidoscope of greens, blues, purples and all the other colours of the rainbow.
3. In the middle of the garden, picture a majestic tree, your Tree of Serenity, a symbol of positivity and everything that you nurture in life.
4. Around the tree, sow more seeds of serenity, each individual seed a metaphor for good things in your life, like forgiveness and self-love.
5. Wander deeper into the garden and visualise the array of flowers, each different one representing more positive aspects of your existence, as you listen to the breeze and birdsong.
6. Picture yourself walking back to the tree, tending it, watering its roots and acknowledging all the positive thoughts in your life. In this mental garden, uproot any weeds, the negative thoughts that hold you back.
7. Feel the deep connection in the garden, and the natural rhythms here, before embracing the velvety darkness of night and sleep.

In essence, the science behind nature's impact on sleep highlights the intricate interplay between our biological systems and the natural world. The good news is your subconscious mind doesn't know the difference between actually being out in the garden or nature versus mentally imagining being there from the comfort of your own bed. If you embrace this concept and commit to practising it regularly, I am confident that you will see a positive shift not only in your sleep patterns but also in your mental health and wellbeing.

10

OUT-OF-BODY SLEEP

Having an out-of-body experience sounds wacky, but trust me when I say that opening your mind to the idea can potentially lead to incredible sleep. I'm going to introduce you to four different Sleep Hacks here, so you can try them all and see which one works best for you.

As ever, you only have to try one Sleep Hack from the Hypnomagical section, in combination with one from each of the Physical and Psychological sections. But read on and prepare to be intrigued …

REALITY AND ILLUSION

In an episode of my 2014 TV3 show *Brainhacker*, I designed an immersive experience that blurred the lines between reality and illusion. At the time I was fascinated by the concept of out-of-body experiences and set out to design a psychological illusion where I would induce an out-of-body experience in myself and use that as a conduit to 'contact the other side'.

Out-of-body experiences are intriguing phenomena in which people perceive themselves as being detached from and floating away from their physical bodies. These experiences have fascinated people for centuries, leading to a multitude of interpretations and explanations across different cultures.

THE *KA* CONCEPT

Many ancient civilisations believed in the existence of a separate soul or spirit that could temporarily leave the body during sleep or trance-like states. For example, in ancient Egypt, the concept of the *ka*, a spiritual double, was central to their beliefs about the afterlife and out-of-body experiences. Similarly, ancient Greek philosophy explored what happened the soul during sleep, as evidenced in the writings of Plato and Aristotle. In indigenous cultures worldwide, out-of-body experiences were often regarded as spiritual moments and were integral to shamanic practices. Shamans believed they could enter altered states of consciousness during rituals or dreams, allowing their spirits to travel to other realms or communicate with ancestors. These experiences were seen as a means of gaining knowledge, healing and spiritual guidance.

For *Brainhacker*, I sought to delve into the mysteries of the human mind in a way that went beyond traditional magic or mentalism. Inspired by the age-old fascination with the afterlife and all things bizarre, I hatched a plan to induce both an out-of-body and a near-death experience for myself, offering viewers a glimpse into the unknown realms that lie beyond the veil.

I assembled an international creative team and we meticulously designed a scenario that would simulate an out-of-body experience under the supervision of a professional medical team. The creative team and I decided (stupidly) it would be amazing to bury me in a tonne of ice in front of a live studio audience which would, coupled with a good dose of self-hypnosis, enable me to have an out-of-body experience. While in this altered state of mind I was hoping to use my skills to contact dead loved ones related to audience members and bring back personal messages from those spirits to those people.

Disclaimer: Although they had no idea how I was doing what I was doing, everyone in the studio was aware that this was a mentalism piece designed for TV and I don't actually believe anyone can actually 'contact the other side'. The studio was designed with moody lighting, mist-filled corridors, and an ambient soundtrack that would heighten the sensory experience.

If you're wondering how all of this is linked to sleep, don't worry, I'll explain shortly!

As the cameras rolled, I was buried in a tonne of ice packed in an ice coffin in front of the live audience. There is no real way to prepare for this. The show was filmed just before my exploration into cold therapy and ice baths and the only real preparation I did was the odd cold shower in advance. Once I was buried in the ice the plan was for me to be in there for around 20 minutes, when, we assumed, I would enter the first stage of hypothermia. Then, using self-hypnosis, I could bring on a state of hallucination that would mirror the stages of a near-death experience.

As the clock ticked something interesting happened. I went to a very deep place in my mind where I had the ability to control my body temperature. Strangely, this had the effect of preventing the very illusion we had designed, as my core temperature remained stable! Twenty minutes passed. Then 25 minutes. After 30 minutes the team got really worried that on the outside I seemed so cold yet very calm. And then a shift happened.

All of a sudden I was transported into a world where I was navigating through a series of strange empty spaces, mimicking the tunnel-like sensations reported by those who have had genuine near-death encounters. Messages came through out of nowhere, which I delivered to audience members who knew in their heart and soul that this information was nothing I could have known in advance, as it was secret information so specific to them. The immersive atmosphere amplified the psychological impact, blurring the lines between reality and illusion.

Having simulated the journey towards the glowing white light at the end of the tunnel, I reached a pivotal moment where the experience transformed from the planned to the unplanned. After 47 minutes, I suddenly went into deep shock and my vital signs lowered. I was in real and unforeseen danger. I was never supposed to have been in the ice coffin for anywhere near this length of time. The medical team intervened and decided I needed to be pulled out immediately. I was still hallucinating and my mind was being hammered with messages from imaginary entities, symbols of the shadowy figures sometimes associated with near death. In their rush to pull me out of the ice coffin the team dropped me, and as my shoulder hit the medical gurney, searing pain went through my whole body. I went into deep shock and started to shake uncontrollably.

It took many hours for the medical team to bring my vital signs back to normal before they released me to return home. That night at home, something happened that I have never spoken about. I fell into a deep, deep sleep until exactly 4.47 a.m. I woke up and sitting at the end of the bed was my deceased granny Lizzie, my mum's mother. She relayed a message to me which she asked me to deliver to my mum, Kitty. I then went to the bathroom and puked for an hour, followed by diarrhoea for another hour.

The next day I told my mum the message Lizzie had passed on. My mum went white as a ghost, as there is no way I could have created or made up this information. For clarity, I do not believe in psychics and I still don't believe it was actually my granny who visited me that night. I cannot explain what happened other than I believe it was me weirdly connecting with a very deep part of my subconscious mind that somehow had that personal information unbeknownst even to me.

For the next 47 days I woke up every night at 4.47 a.m. with cold sweats, followed by more puking and diarrhoea. I'm not superstitious at all, but I was freaking out that the number 47 was haunting me. On the 48th day I went to the doctor and got bloodwork done. I was really scared I might have done some permanent damage to myself. Thankfully my body began to return back to normal that day and my bloodwork results came back all clear on 21 December – they were stamped, strangely, with the time 4.47 p.m. The medical team's opinion is that my kidneys had suffered as a result of being in the ice for so long but that over the following days and weeks they had slowly recuperated.

The simulated out-of-body/near-death experience for *Brainhacker* was a crazy idea that was meant to push the boundaries of entertainment and exploration. I've done a lot of crazy and truly dangerous stunts over the years but this is the one I honestly regret doing, as it really messed with my mind and body, and, indeed, my sleep. It made me think deeply about the nature of perception, the power of suggestion, and the age-old quest to understand what lies beyond this life.

While the episode was a captivating journey, it also served as a reminder of the responsibility that comes with manipulating perceptions. It highlighted the fine line between entertainment and ethical considerations, emphasising the importance of transparency when delving into topics as profound as the afterlife.

So here's the rub – during those weeks I was sick I tried everything to sleep, but I still woke up every single night, scared and sick. And then I had an epiphany. What if I could use this experience as inspiration to design a new method for attaining deep sleep?

After some trial and error, I landed on the following Out-of-Body Sleep script. I began to use it when I was still waking in the middle of the night and it fixed my sleep 100 per cent. I stopped waking up in the middle of the night and slept soundly by using it. I use it now specifically when I want to dissociate my mind from my body and forget about everything and everyone in my life. I use it when I want to become an empty vessel prepared for sleep. Colleagues and clients of mine have also used it with great success.

Although the above true story may seem extreme and scary, it is important for you to know that at various moments in my life I have had troubles with my sleep, and although the following was designed as a direct result of what happened in *Brainhacker*, I can assure you there is nothing scary or frightening about the technique that resulted from the experience.

SLEEP HACK 18
OUT-OF-BODY SLEEP

An audio recording where I guide you through this visualisation can be accessed on my website www.keithbarry.com/sleephacks with the password SLEEPHACKS24.

> Lie down in your bed, close your eyes, take a deep breath in, and then exhale super slowly until your lungs are completely empty. Do this 10 times. Take some time to focus on your breath, and with each breath you inhale allow yourself to fully relax in preparation for deep sleep.
> Become aware of your body and how it feels. Imagine your body becoming weightless, as though you are gently levitating, as if by magic, above your bed. Take some time to really visualise this and get a sense of the freedom of your spirit, liberated now from the confines of your physical form.
> Next, imagine your body floating out of the levitating physical version of yourself. Visualise this entity as your *ka*, floating effortlessly towards your ceiling. Floating and drifting, drifting and floating. Repeat the following silently to yourself 50 times: 'I am free to float and drift, drift and float.'
> Now imagine you can see yourself from the *ka* version of yourself floating from above. Look at how peaceful you are at this exact moment in your bed. Notice that this version of you at this exact moment is a version of you so peaceful and calm that you are ready for deep sleep. See the details of your bedsheets from above. The colours, the wrinkles in not only your sheets but your face. If you notice any tension or

wrinkles in your face or body from your floating version of yourself, allow those parts to relax and smooth out.

- Allow any tension or worries you have to release from your physical form up and into your *ka* floating form. Picture those tensions and worries as shapes, words and entities exiting like a gentle mist from your mind and being absorbed into the mind and body of your ethereal form. Take a few moments until you are sure you have projected all your worries and concerns onto and into that spiritual *ka* version of yourself.
- Embrace the sense of lightness and calmness that now begins to permeate your entire physical being. Take a moment to enjoy this imagined out-of-body experience and allow yourself to drift and float into a deep state of wonderful relaxation.
- When you notice a sense of lightness and calmness, imagine the floating version of yourself dissolving away and disappearing into the night sky.
- Repeat the following mantra silently over and over to yourself: 'My mind is quiet and my body is at peace.'
- If you find your mind wandering from your mantra, just gently remind yourself to return to it until you enter into a deep sleep.

TRY THIS: THE POWER OF COLD Cold therapy seems all the rage now. Before it became a trend, my ice coffin experiment all those years ago inspired me to look into the benefits of cold therapy. People all over the world are currently posting videos of themselves in freezing cold ice baths, as popularised by the iceman, Wim Hof. I am also a fan of cold therapy and take ice baths almost every day. I know that most of you reading this will either have no interest in taking an ice bath or could not be bothered with the hassle of it all. But there is a cold therapy hack that can serve as a sleep aid. I challenge you to take a freezing cold shower for two minutes every single morning for the next year. If you take a cold shower in the morning it will dump a healthy level of cortisol, adrenaline and serotonin into your body, which will in turn help regulate your circadian rhythm. Start by having your shower as normal and then turning the water to freezing cold for ten seconds at the end. Add on five seconds daily until you reach two minutes. Do that every day for a year and then send me an email with the results!

REMOTE VIEWING SLEEP

Another concept I find fascinating and have researched extensively is the idea of remote viewing. It's a so-called psychic ability that involves somehow remotely seeing a distant or unseen target, typically a place, written document or future event, using extrasensory perception (ESP). The idea of remote viewing was explored by the US government in the 1970s and 1980s. In the Stargate Project the CIA used people who claimed psychic ability in order to discover classified information about rival countries.

The person with the supposed ability to engage in remote viewing is known as the viewer. These people claim to be able to perceive details about a target by using a heightened sense of intuition or even a claimed sixth sense. Many times the viewer would go into an altered state of mind using self-hypnosis in order to achieve the desired result. A target would be set for the viewer – this would be a specific location or classified documents that the viewer is attempting to describe. It is often selected by an independent party other than the viewer to eliminate bias.

Many remote viewing experiments involve a blind or even double blind element, meaning that the viewer does not know anything other than the most basic target information; they don't know any details about the target in advance of the session. This helps to eliminate the possibility of subconscious bias influencing the remote viewing event. During a remote viewing session, the viewer often produces sketches, written descriptions, or oral accounts of the perceived target.

It's important to note that the scientific community, including myself, remains sceptical about the validity of remote viewing. While some research studies claim positive results, others argue that methodological flaws and biases could explain any apparent success. Remote viewing falls outside the mainstream scientific understanding of perception and communication, and it is generally considered a pseudoscience by the majority of the scientific community.

The Stargate Project was eventually terminated due to a lack of concrete evidence supporting the practical application of remote viewing for intelligence purposes. Despite this, remote viewing continues to be a topic of interest in certain paranormal and New Age communities. I also genuinely believe that many countries around the world are still running projects like the Stargate Project – we will only find out about these projects when they are either declassified or a whistle-blower exposes them.

Several remote viewing experiments were conducted as part of the Stargate Project, and some of them gained attention for their intriguing results. One of the most intriguing examples was Joseph McMoneagle, who claimed to have remote viewed a crashed Soviet Tu-22 bomber in Africa during one of his sessions. Some argued that the details provided were accurate, while sceptics questioned the consistency and reliability of such information.

There are many stories involving viewers remote viewing top secret vaults in other countries and landmines during the Vietnam War, and more recently they have apparently been used to locate oil for oil mining companies. Again, to be super clear, I personally take all these claims with a pinch of salt.

The reason I provide you with this background information is because this was the inspiration behind a mentalism demonstration I did nightly during my *Dark Side* tour in 2013, which led to an amazing discovery that we will use shortly as a sleep aid.

Every night on stage I would hypnotise someone on a hospital gurney and have them remote view into a sealed envelope which was hanging above the stage. They would wake up with details and images that would accurately describe a photograph that I had sealed inside the envelope in advance of the show. I discovered that an unexpected side effect was occurring nightly. Almost every night, with the hypnotic language I was using to induce trance, the participants fell into deep delta brainwave sleep, instead of an alpha brainwave state, which is what I needed in order to accomplish the effect. I used this as the catalyst to begin exploring this language with people who were having difficulty sleeping and had some amazing results. The technique is as follows.

SLEEP HACK 19
REMOTE VIEWING VISUALISATION

An audio recording where I guide you through this visualisation can be accessed on my website www.keithbarry.com/sleephacks with the password SLEEPHACKS24.

> Decide on a relaxing target location for this remote viewing visualisation. It could be a butterfly farm, a beautiful, quiet Japanese garden, a sky filled with hot air balloons, or any other imagined location you think you would find super relaxing. Our aim here is to quickly achieve a deep delta brainwave state of mind. Take some time to decide what type of relaxing target would suit you and quickly sketch out the target on a piece of paper. Place this piece of paper under your pillow.

> Lie down, close your eyes and take a long, deep breath in and out. Before you imagine yourself remote viewing, begin by visualising yourself in an isolated canyon, far away from the business of everyday life. See yourself reclining in a specially designed acoustic hammock, where you become immersed in an extraordinary auditory experience that transcends the boundaries of the ordinary.

> Imagine the hammock rocking you gently, suspended between the canyon walls, and beneath you, the orange, sandy ground gradually descends into the depths of the gorge. The air is a soft, gentle breeze, and a serene atmosphere envelops the canyon, making it the perfect sanctuary for relaxation and remote viewing.

> Now envision the hammock itself as more than just a comfortable resting place; it channels the soothing vibrations

and calming vibes of the natural surroundings. As you settle into the hammock, using your imagination you begin to notice a subtle, rhythmic vibration that emerges from the very heart of the canyon. These gentle vibrations are like the heartbeat of the Earth itself, creating a wonderful atmosphere that tunes in with the very essence of the surroundings. Take some time to truly imagine this and to align your own heartbeat with the gentle heartbeat of the Earth.

> Listen for any calming sounds that echo through the canyon walls. The rustle of leaves, the distant murmur of a meandering stream, and the soft calls of an eagle create a beautiful harmonious atmosphere. The soundwaves bounce off the rocky surfaces, creating a unique acoustic tapestry that swirls around you. Take time to really imagine this.

> Allow the hushed whispers of nature to permeate every fibre of your being, creating a sensation of being cradled not just by the hammock but by the very vibrations of the canyon itself.

> As the vibrations continue, pay attention to the gentle frequency of the canyon's soundwaves, each curve of the rock contributing to the complex interplay of sound. This unique auditory experience transcends the ordinary, transporting you to a state of profound relaxation and connection with the natural world.

> Now, as you lie relaxed in the hammock in your imagination, call out 'It's time to sleep', and hear the echo of those words bouncing off the walls of the canyon. If you think about this logically the sound will bounce indefinitely in the walls as it echoes back and forth from one end to the other. Listen

to the sound of your voice echoing 'It's time to sleep' for as long as you like.

› In this tranquil haven, as you drift and float in your hammock, the canyon becomes a portal to a realm where you can begin to let go of reality and remote view your chosen target.

› Take time now to float out of the canyon towards your chosen target location for deep relaxation. Allow yourself to bask and bathe in this imagined experience. Really make every effort to make this target place your new reality. Allow your brainwave state to slow down in unison to align with what you are visualising as your target to aid you in your quest to sleep.

› Stay in and explore this place until you gently nod off into the target itself, enjoying every single moment of wonderful relaxation as it happens.

VIRTUAL REALITY

The current state of virtual reality (VR) technology allows people to enter into a world of escapism that temporarily detaches them from the physical world. VR headsets, with their ability to transport users into a virtual world, provide an escape into an alternative universe. We will use the principle of VR technology as a springboard into deep sleep. Remember, your mind does not know the difference between something imagined and reality, so you can create your own virtual world by using your imagination instead of investing large sums of money on a VR headset. Instead of the headset you only need your mind. And your mind is free!

The conscious use of your imagination as if you are wearing a VR headset allows for a gentle disconnection from the challenges of the waking world, paving the way for an organic and rejuvenating sleep experience.

SLEEP HACK 20
VIRTUAL REALITY VISUALISATION

An audio recording where I guide you through this visualisation can be accessed on my website www.keithbarry.com/sleephacks with the password SLEEPHACKS24.

> - Lie in your bed, close your eyes and imagine that you have just strapped on your brand new VR headset. This imagined headset is super special, as it will allow you to step into the realm of your own mind with the aid of virtual reality, imagining a journey that takes you deep into the intricate landscapes of your mind.
> - As you immerse yourself in the virtual reality experience, start by visualising the unique brainwave frequencies of your brain and what they might look like. Picture yourself as a tiny stickperson surfing these brainwaves, gliding effortlessly through the neural connections and intricate internal circuitry inside your mind.
> - As you ride the crest of your brainwaves, observe the vibrant bursts of energy that signify brainwave activity. Allow the gentle roll of the waves of your mind to guide you into a state of profound detachment, separating from the external world and immersing yourself within the depths of your own consciousness.

> Navigate through the terrain of your mind, passing through regions associated with anxiety and stress. Visualise these brainwaves fading away, like a wave in the sea fading as it hits the shore, as you journey deeper into the inner recesses and workings of your mind. Imagine each new brainwave as a burst of vibrant colour as you encounter pockets of creativity and imagination, providing a detailed blueprint of your inner mental sanctuary.

> Imagine your awareness blending with the soothing hum of your brain's electrical signals, creating a seamless flow of soothing soundwaves that resonate throughout the network of your mind. Explore and surf the brainwaves of relaxation, and feel a sense of liberation from the confines of your physical body, allowing the virtual reality experience to guide you into a state of profound calmness.

> Your imagined virtual reality headset will become a portal to the inner recesses of your mind, where you can access a deep neurological place that goes beyond the boundaries of everyday stress. Be sure to explore this area for an extended period of time as you prepare for sleep. Let the immersive experience pave the way for a restful and rejuvenating night's sleep, as your brainwaves gently carry you into the realm of dreams, leaving behind the concerns of the waking world.

FLOTATION THERAPY

On another episode of my TV3 show *Brainhacker*, I performed an effect I'd dreamed of doing for years. The Crimmins triplets, who are influencers in the beauty industry, were invited on my show, entitled *Intuition*, in order to test them for extrasensory abilities.

Using a strategy very similar to remote viewing, I placed them into a sleepy altered state of mind and asked them to imagine I had a tattoo. I asked them to stare at my bare arm and describe what the tattoo might look like inside their minds.

They described a tattoo involving an eye, a clock and the word 'extraordinary'. I then asked them, 'What if that tattoo is not only in your mind? What if that's a tattoo I've already got?' They looked bemused and confused. I then took a wet wipe to my arm and began to rub. A tattoo slowly started to appear. A tattoo that matched the tattoo they had just designed in their mind. It was actually a real tattoo that the make-up artist had perfectly camouflaged backstage by spraying over it with make-up that matched the colour of my arm. I then showed video footage of me getting the tattoo a week before we recorded the episode to the triplets. Needless to say, they were astonished, as was the rest of the studio audience.

Here's the crazy thing. The tattoo was designed and done by an amazing tattoo artist called Joe Myler, who has sadly since passed away. He was dumbfounded himself to see that during each sitting (the tattoo is a half sleeve, so it took three sittings) I fell asleep. The reason this was unusual is because most people wince the whole way through due to the pain of getting a tattoo. I fell asleep every single time.

In the weeks running up to getting the tattoo, I had explored flotation therapy. This is where you relax in a flotation tank where you can't hear or see anything. Technically, this is known as restricted environment stimulation therapy (REST). It allows you to enter a state of deep relaxation, and induces a meditative calmness of the mind. REST has been shown in studies to reduce stress, alleviate muscle tension, pain and depression and improve mood.[38]

You can use flotation therapy as a springboard into the following visualisation that you can use anytime, anywhere, without the need for an expensive tank.

SLEEP HACK 21
SENSORY DEPRIVATION TANK

An audio recording where I guide you through this visualisation can be accessed on my website www.keithbarry.com/sleephacks with the password SLEEPHACKS24.

> Close your eyes, lie down, take a deep breath in and out and imagine yourself in a serene and tranquil space. Visualise a room painted in soft, warm colours, with gentle atmospheric orange lighting that soothes your senses. The air is pleasantly warm, creating a cocoon of comfort around you.
> In the centre of the room is a sleek, silver, futuristic pod – a sensory deprivation tank designed to transport you to a realm of unparalleled relaxation. Approach the tank in your mind with a sense of anticipation, feeling the coolness of the air against your skin.
> As you open the lid of the tank, a subtle hiss escapes, releasing a cloud of warm steam that gently envelops you. Lie down in the tank, allowing the water inside to surround your body. The buoyancy and temperature of the water induce an immediate sense of weightlessness.
> As you recline in the buoyant water, feel the silky smoothness against your skin. The tank is filled with a solution of Epsom salts, dissolving tension, promoting healing and a profound sense of weightless suspension. Gradually allow yourself to

float effortlessly on the surface, trusting the water to support you completely.

- Allow the lid of the tank to close down, shutting out any external noises or stimuli. The soft, diffused blue light inside begins to fade, casting the interior into a gentle darkness. Embrace the quietness as the world outside disappears, replaced only by the rhythmic sound of your own breath.
- The sensory deprivation tank is designed to immerse you in silence, allowing your mind to relax and unwind. As you float and drift, imagine the gentle ebb and flow of your breath synchronising with the gentle movement of the water around you. Sense the boundaries between your body and the liquid environment blurring until they become one. It's almost like your body is melting into the fluid that surrounds you.
- Visualise the absence of any senses now as a canvas for your mind to paint its own tranquil scene. Perhaps you envision a serene beach, with soft waves lapping at the shore, or a peaceful forest with leaves gently rustling in the breeze. Allow your mind to wander without any of the pressures of the external world.
- With each passing moment, feel the tension dissolve from your muscles. Your mind, which just moments ago was whizzing and whirring with thoughts, begins to drift into a state of profound calmness. The sensory deprivation tank becomes a portal for mental clarity and deep relaxation, an escape from the noise of everyday life.

I have described several techniques here for you to try. Remember, you don't have to do all of them, and you only have to select one to combine with your chosen Physical and Psychological Sleep Hacks for the first 30 days. But I recommend trying all of them at least once. The feeling of being out of your body can be transformative, and it goes without saying that it's deeply relaxing.

11

CLOSING QUESTIONS

As you come to the end of the book, I am confident that if you try the techniques I've described you will find your sleep improving. Remember, it's all about finding what works for you, as well as the necessary discipline of sticking to your chosen three of the 21 Sleep Hacks, one from each of the three sections – Physical, Psychological and Hypnomagical – for at least 30 days. If this particular combination isn't working for you, swap one out. Keep swapping until you come across your own, personal, unique winning formula, which I am confident that you will.

The 'Try This' suggestions are just that – only suggestions. They're not essential to your success, whereas the three Sleep Hacks from each section are non-negotiables. But I would also heavily encourage you to give some of them a shot because you might find them super effective.

SOME QUESTIONS YOU MAY HAVE
HOW SOON SHOULD I SEE AN IMPROVEMENT IN MY SLEEP?

The timeline for improvement varies from person to person. Some people will see immediate improvement; for others it may take up to 30 days or longer. Patience is crucial, as rewiring your brain for better sleep can take some time.

WHAT IF I DON'T SEE AN IMPROVEMENT IN MY SLEEP AND THE BOOK'S TECHNIQUES DON'T WORK FOR ME?

I am confident that if you follow the plan outlined in the book you should see an improvement. The key is to find a combination of techniques that works for you. Trial and error are essential and tweaking the different techniques so they suit you is also recommended. NGU – Never Give Up – until you find that combination that does work for you! If you really find that nothing is working, consider finding a sleep specialist to work with one-to-one in order to help resolve any ongoing issues.

I CAN FALL ASLEEP, BUT I KEEP WAKING UP IN THE MIDDLE OF THE NIGHT AND THEN I CAN'T FALL BACK TO SLEEP. WHAT CAN I DO?

This happens to me regularly and is more common than one might think. I'll start by stating what you should not do. Do not open your phone! Do not turn on the TV! Do not pace around the house! Instead, use your favourite self-hypnosis technique from the book to settle yourself back into a deep sleep.

I SOMETIMES DO SHIFT WORK, WHICH PLAYS HAVOC WITH MY SLEEP. DO YOU HAVE ANY ADVICE ABOUT WHAT I CAN DO?

Setting a regular sleep schedule is key. I know shift work can be tricky, but establishing a sleep schedule, even on your days off, really will help. If you do find you're wrecked when you are supposed to be awake and alert, strategic napping really can help. I recommend 15 minutes' napping with a blindfold on while listening to soothing music with binaural beats. This is what I personally do when I'm on a crazy travel schedule and I find it works wonders for my energy levels.

MY PARTNER SNORES AND WAKES ME UP. IS IT TIME FOR SEPARATE ROOMS?

This is a difficult one to answer, as the science is split on this. While it may be a temporary solution, I believe the benefits of intimacy and the release of feel-good hormones such as oxytocin from sleeping with your partner outweigh the downside of them snoring. If your partner snores you can ask them to try some solutions such as nasal strips, an anti-snoring mouthpiece or sleeping on their side. Alternatively, you can try using a good set of noise-cancelling earplugs, which should drown out their snoring.

CAN SEX HELP ME SLEEP BETTER AT NIGHT?

A healthy sex life can absolutely help with your sleep. Studies show that sex can help improve sleep, but only if you achieve an orgasm.[39] Have you ever had a better incentive to improve your sex life and ensure you climax?

I HAVE PROBLEMS VISUALISING. CAN YOU RECOMMEND HOW TO GET BETTER AT IT?

When I meet people who have difficulty visualising, I encourage them to simply imagine they can visualise. By imagining you can visualise you will eventually become better at it. Also be sure to engage all the senses when visualising – taste, touch, smell, sight and sound. I'm also a huge fan of doodling to create a visual representation of what you are attempting to visualise. Start simple and then as you progress your doodles can become more intricate. For example, if you are trying the Sleepscape Garden technique, you can doodle what that would look like in advance of your visualisation. This will serve as a mental bridge between reality and your imagination and it is a great way to help focus the mind.

HOW DO I DEAL WITH JETLAG?

This is something I have to contend with regularly and I know how debilitating it can be. What's worked best for me is adjusting my sleep schedule before departure, using light exposure, and also avoiding napping in the new time zone.

IF MY SLEEP IS IMPROVING BUT I STILL HAVE SOME BAD NIGHTS, WHAT'S THE BEST WAY TO RECOVER THE MORNING AFTERWARDS?

First and foremost, be kind to yourself! Seriously, don't beat yourself up. It happens to all of us. When it happens, I recommend you get some sunlight and do some light exercise, but try not to overdo the exercise. Don't overdo the coffee, as this will have a detrimental effect on your next night's sleep. Ensure you are properly hydrated and, if you need to, take a 15-minute nap. A good nap can really help when you are struggling after a disturbed night's sleep.

WHAT'S THE MOST OUTLANDISH SLEEP MYTH YOU'VE ENCOUNTERED WHILE RESEARCHING FOR THIS BOOK?

It's a complete myth that you can 'catch up' on lost sleep. Do not think of sleep as a bank that you can replenish at weekends. Instead of digging into your sleep overdraft, always keep some credits in your sleep account!

*

I really hope the insights I've shared in this book ignite an appreciation inside you for the power of sleep and the ability you have to control and harness that power. By harnessing the mysteries of sleep, you will unlock the extraordinary untapped potential of your subconscious mind and potentially add years to your life. Wishing you the sweetest of dreams and a life full of energy and positivity.

– KB

12

JUST FOR CHILDREN!

The following story is designed to be read at night-time to your child when they are in bed and preparing to sleep. There is hypnotic language embedded into the story which will create an atmosphere of relaxation in readiness for sleep. Feel free to play with and change the story as time progresses, but follow the guidelines below to have the most impact and the highest chance of your child falling asleep.

1. Words in italics are to be said in a gentle, soothing manner which will induce a sense of calmness and will subliminally encourage your child to relax.
2. Where you see (**P**), pause for five seconds. There are deliberate pause points throughout the story. These pause points will help your child to absorb your suggestions subconsciously and

induce a sleepy state of mind. If you see multiple (**P**)s, add them together and pause for that length of time.
3. Be sure to use a smooth and steady rhythm throughout. A hypnotist's voice maintains a steady and unhurried pace. This will help guide your child's mind towards a receptive and relaxed state.
4. You may notice some words being repeated. This is deliberate, as we want to reinforce the suggestion of sleep throughout the story.
5. It may take some time for the story to have an effect. Be sure to commit to telling the story every night for at least 30 nights in order to assess its effectiveness. Of course, only tell the story if your child is truly enjoying it and engaging with the process.

SAMMY'S SNOOZEVILLE SUPERPOWER

Once upon a time there was a 14-year-old boy from the town of *Yawnville* named Sammy. He was tall for his age, six feet two inches to be exact, and although he looked perfectly normal he was actually a teenager who hid an amazing secret. *His extraordinary ability was being able to put anyone to sleep, any time, anywhere, using something called hypnosis.* Hypnosis is where a friendly person called a hypnotist has a special talent where they can use gentle words *to guide you into relaxation and sleep, with no worries or fears.* Sometimes when you are in this *sleepy state* a hypnotist can ignite your imagination and help you achieve your goals and dreams. The hypnotist can also use hypnosis to help you overcome fears, worries and anxiety and any other problems you might have inside your mind.

When someone is in hypnosis it's almost like *floating on a giant fluffy cloud* (**P**), where you are so *comfortable and calm* that you just want to *chill out, relax and go into a deep, deep sleep* **(P)**. In that state of mind you become suggestible – which means that whatever the hypnotist says or suggests to you becomes your new reality. It's almost like being inside a virtual reality machine. Except there are no batteries or power needed because the machine exists inside your mind!

On his 14th birthday his parents surprised Sammy with a trip to Edinburgh in Scotland to visit the famous castle there. As he was walking through the streets of Edinburgh he discovered a magic shop full of amazing magic tricks – it was a treasure trove of colourful boxes, magic wands, wizardry gadgets and illusions which were spread throughout the shop, but what captured Sammy's attention was the library of books, both old and new, sitting on shelves that seemed to float as if by magic in the back of the shop **(PP)**.

Sammy had spent two hours browsing through the books when one book really caught his eye – *Hypnosis for the Complete Klutz*. He was fascinated to discover in the book some new hypnosis techniques that his mentor Tony Sadar had not shared with him. Sammy bought the book for £15 and brought it back to the Grand Hotel, where he and his family were staying.

As night-time arrived and the sun set Sammy got ready for bed. He brushed his teeth, put on his comfy PJs, said goodnight to his parents and his sister Michelle and crawled into bed, exhausted with tiredness from the long day exploring Edinburgh.

But, as tired as he was, with his eyes getting heavier and heavier, and his muscles getting more and more loose and relaxed, he began to read this mysterious book on hypnosis, sleep and relaxation underneath the bed covers **(P)**.

He discovered that by just using his words he could not only get people to go into a *deep sleep* and help them achieve their goals and dreams, he could also get them to become the stars of a stage show where they would do anything he asked them to do, always with their permission, of course.

He began to imagine what it would feel like to be on a stage in a theatre in front of an audience of thousands with dozens of people on stage *deeply asleep* under his hypnotic spell. He learned the power of words and how *right now, in just a single moment*, he could put someone into a *deep sleep* **(P)**.

His sister Michelle had problems sleeping, so he practised on her by saying:

'Your eyes are beginning to get heavier and heavier, your heart rate is starting to slow down, your muscles are beginning to relax, that's it, relaxing every muscle, nerve and fibre in your body. Your toes are relaxed, your ankles, your shins, your knees, your calf muscles, your legs are getting heavier and heavier, your stomach muscles, your chest, your neck, your shoulders, your head, your arms, your back are getting loose and relaxed. Your back muscles are softening. Your whole body now is so deeply relaxed it just wants to go to sleep' **(PP)**.

He could see Michelle's body was getting more and more relaxed, deeply relaxed just as you are now.

He continued talking to Michelle:

'Now imagine a sunbeam touching your face and all the tension leaving your body **(P)**. *When I count backwards from ten you'll find you just drift away into a nice, calm, deep sleep* **(P)**.

Ten – you are happy, healthy and sleepy **(P)**

Nine – you are confident, brave and sleepy **(P)**

Eight – you are wonderful, talented and sleepy **(P)**

Seven – you are kind, generous, and sleepy **(P)**

Six – you are creative, strong and sleepy **(P)**

Five – you are friendly, positive, and sleepy **(P)**

Four – you are honest, caring and sleepy **(P)**

Three – you are magical, respectful and sleepy **(P)**

Two – you are funny, adventurous and sleepy **(P)**

One – you are relaxed, calm and sleepy **(P)**

Yesterday is gone, tomorrow is a new day. Right here, right now, nothing matters except deep, deep, sleep **(P)**.'

And just like a magic trick Michelle had *drifted off into a nice deep sleep*. Sammy couldn't believe it. He decided then and there that he was going to become the world's greatest hypnotist.

He soon realised that almost anyone can be hypnotised. You see, you just need three things. Imagination, intelligence and the ability to *fall into sleep – three things which you also have. Try this. Close your eyes if they are not already closed. Take a nice, long, soothing deep breath in and out and allow your mind and body to relax.* Now try not to imagine a blue giraffe in a pink dress dancing on its head **(P)**. If you just saw a blue giraffe in a pink dress dancing on its head it means you have a great imagination and you can use that imagination to achieve anything you want in life.

Now answer this silently in your mind – what's one plus one? If you got two as the answer, congratulations, you have intelligence. And we all know you have the third thing – *the ability to sleep deeply*. If you were with Sammy *now*, he could put you *into a nice, deep, soothing sleep at this exact moment*. Where all *your worries would just fade away*, and you would dream a beautiful dream where you would see all the things you want to do in life as a perfect movie *inside your sleepy mind* **(PP)**.

Within a year of buying that book, Sammy was on the biggest indoor stage in Ireland, the 3Arena. Eight thousand people were in the audience. He asked the entire audience to clasp their two hands together tightly and to imagine superglue between their hands. Then he snapped his fingers and said the words *'sleep deeply now'*. Sure enough, all eight thousand people fell into a deep hypnotic spell. Sammy was amazed at the sight of all these people slumped over in their seats snoring and drooling in a really deep sleep. It was just over a year since he read his first book on hypnosis and now eight thousand people were fast asleep!

He wanted to have an amazing impact on them all, so instead of beginning the show by getting them to act out funny things like clucking like a chicken or imagining they were aliens he decided to gift them all *the ability to get rid of their noisy and annoying thoughts and be able to go into a tranquil, deep sleep every single night* (**P**).

With your eyes closed as you *get ready to sleep soundly tonight*, follow along now with what Sammy said to the audience: *Relax your body and sink and melt down and just drift away* (**P**). *Drift away into a nice calm, deep sleep* (**P**). *Deeper and deeper, sleepier and sleepier you go* (**P**). *Deeper and deeper you go, and with every word that I say and even the spaces between my words you find you drift away even deeper towards a lovely calm night's sleep* (**P**).

Now in your mind imagine you are holding a bottle of magical bubbles (**PP**). Every time you blow a bubble it will be a different colour representing a different worry, fear or concern you might have. Imagine now you blow a bubble – it's coloured red. See your concern or worry inside the bubble. Maybe it's a word you see. Maybe it's a place or a face. Know now that you are safe blowing this bubble and nothing and no one can harm you. Now see that bubble *floating and drifting* higher and higher and higher into the night sky towards the stars above **(P)**. See it floating so far away that you can barely see it. Now you see it pop and vanish into thin air. Now blow another bubble, this time a purple one. See a different worry inside this bubble. Again, see the bubble *floating and drifting* higher and higher away. *Drifting and floating, floating and drifting. Yesterday is gone, tomorrow is a new day. Right here, right now, nothing matters except pure relaxation* and that bubble floating so high that whatever worry it contains doesn't bother you anymore and it simply pops, and along with it your worry vanishes too. Do this with different-coloured bubbles and worries in silence, with your eyes closed, for the next ten seconds **(PP)**.

Fantastic. The audience watching Sammy did this too. They felt *more confident than they had ever felt before* and they knew they had *the power to vanish* their problems *instantly and also get a good, long night's sleep whenever they wanted* **(P)**.

They were now ready to be entertained by Sammy. He brought a hundred people on stage and immediately *put them back to sleep*. He suggested to them that they would all believe they were members of an orchestra, with each person playing a different instrument. Upon his command they played imaginary trumpets, saxophones, drums, guitars, violins and any number of other imaginary instruments **(PP)**.

He then suggested they would all believe they were on the world's biggest rollercoaster with 247 loop-the-loops. They screamed the wildest of screams and laughed the loudest of laughs as the imaginary rollercoaster twisted and turned at the fastest of speeds in their minds **(P)**.

The funniest things happened, with people even believing their mouth was on their forehead, and when Sammy's assistants gave them ice cream cones they smashed them over and over again on their heads, thinking that's where they should be eating the ice creams. The ice cream dripped down their smiley faces as the rest of the audience howled with laughter **(P)**.

After two hours of performing Sammy put them to *sleep again* one final time. *Sleep deep, deeper and deeper, sleepier and sleepier, right here, right now, in this moment nothing matters except deep sleep, he said* **(P)**. He now suggested to them that they would be *sleepy superheroes*, who could only save the day by using objects and things related to *sleep*.

One person tried to fly with an imaginary bedsheet. Another used an imaginary teddy bear as a villain-fighting tool. Another used an imaginary hot water bottle to be a firefighting hero putting out a fiery baddie **(PP)**!

As the show was coming to a hilarious end, with a hundred people believing they were *sleepy superheroes*, something very strange happened. They all *began to fall asleep* on stage without Sammy saying the words *sleep, deep now* **(P)**. Each and every person *yawned* as they *drifted away into a peaceful slumber*. There was no reason for them to *fall asleep* and Sammy looked confused. He tried to wake them up but couldn't. They were all safe and calm but *fast asleep* on stage *now*. The audience were astounded, as it looked amazing until Sammy explained it wasn't part of the show and he couldn't wake them up!

He then saw a shadow of a person exiting through a fire exit at the back of the theatre. Although the person was far away he recognised them. He knew that walk, that posture, but most important he recognised that walking stick. It was his number one rival, a hypnotist who had copied Sammy for years, The Great Maldini. That was his stage name, but his real name was far more ordinary – Alan Byrnes. Alan and Sammy had gone to school together and had been best friends for years until Alan stole Sammy's book *Hypnosis for the Complete Klutz*. Sammy realised that Alan had stolen the book, and although he did get it back it was too late. Alan had photocopied the book and learned all its hypnotic and *sleepy* secrets. He invented the stage name The Great Maldini and began performing in competition with Sammy. He also hired a mentor, Mesmera the Amazing, who was known as the best female hypnotist the world had ever seen. Alan was a good hypnotist but never as good as Sammy. He was always stealing Sammy's ideas and routines and performing them badly in his own show.

But Alan also had a secret – Mesmera the Amazing had gifted him a top secret piece of technology called a Snoozeslumber 2000. It was secretly hidden inside the walking stick. It resembled a tuning fork that one might use to tune a piano, mixed with some very sophisticated technology. It hid the power of a special *sleep* sound, which was a rare and mythical sound that Mesmera had invented to *send people to dreamland*. The walking stick was also a directional sound speaker, which meant the sound emitted could only be heard by the people the stick was pointed at. When it was pointed at the people on stage they had an irresistible urge to *snuggle into a cosy slumber*. The people on stage had *drifted off to the Land of Nod, where they began to dream as if they were in a field of fluffy feathers* (**P**).

Sammy knew he must find Alan, as the only way to break this *sleepy* spell was to use the high-pitched frequency from the Snoozeslumber 2000 – in other words a super-squeaky sound that would wake up anyone from any sleep or hypnotic spell.

The audience quietly exited the theatre and Sammy made sure the *sleeping* subjects on stage were *comfortable and calm*. He and his team placed pillows underneath everyone's heads and put on a calming lullaby, woven with musical notes that danced like drowsy fireflies, which created an *irresistible urge* for the people *to drift even deeper into a cosy slumber* **(PP)**.

He then ran as fast as his legs could carry him to the one place he knew for certain he would find Alan. The *Zenflo Hypnolagoon*.

The *Zenflo Hypnolagoon* is a *mesmerising and magical* flotation tank designed to transport people into a place of *calm, deep relaxation*. From the outside it looks like a mini UFO, a sphere surrounded by blue LED lights and any number of electrical buttons and controls. Once you step inside you are greeted by a spacious interior filled with lukewarm salty water and *deeply relaxing music* **(P)**.

As you lie down and float weightlessly, all your problems and issues seem to just drift away **(P)**. People who float like this are transformed into another world as the *Zenflo* technology synchronises the lights and sounds inside with the person's *soft breathing and gentle heartbeat*. Imagine now what it might be like to enter into the Zenflo Hypnolagoon and notice how relaxed, calm and peaceful it feels to just float and drift away. Keep floating and drifting in silence for the next ten seconds **(P)**.

Now back to our story. Sammy arrived at the lagoon looking for Alan. The problem was there were ten *Zenflos*, all closed, with people inside. While Sammy was sure Alan was there he couldn't tell which *Zenflo* he was in.

Sammy had an idea. He did something no one should ever do, but he had a responsibility to the people on stage in the theatre to return them back to normal. So he hit the emergency fire button. Alarms rang loudly and the blue fire lights in the ceiling spun wildly. People ran out of their *Zenflos* soaking wet in their swimwear, still half asleep, *yawning* yet running out the door. All of the *Zenflos* emptied. All except one.

Sammy approached with caution. He hit the Open button on the outside of the *Zenflo* and as it opened he saw a horrid yet hilarious sight. Alan was *floating* inside, wearing pink swimming togs and a bright yellow swim cap and clutching a purple rubber chicken (**P**). *His eyes were closed*, and he had a blissful grin on his face. He had *drifted off* into a world of whimsical *dreams*. Sammy asked him, while he was still in hypnosis and *fast asleep*, where the *Snoozeslumber* 2000 was. He got no response. But he had a hack. A brain hack that he knew would work. He decided to put Alan into a *dream within a dream, a hypnotic spell within a hypnotic spell, a float within a float*, and then ask him where the *Snoozeslumber* was.

Sammy used the words: 'As you sleep deeply now and drift and float away swiftly you will accept that everything I say will become your new reality. You will feel as I ask you to feel and think as I ask you to think, and answer any questions I may have for you honestly and sincerely. *Allow yourself to float even deeper in this moment, right here, right now, nothing matters except my voice and wonderful relaxation* (**P**).'

He then asked: 'Where is the *Snoozeslumber* 2000 that *you* used to put all the people into a *deep sleep*, enchanted by your spell?'

After a long pause that seemed like an eternity, Alan, while still *asleep* in a hypnotic trance, responded: 'It's inside my yellow swim cap, of course.' Sammy couldn't believe that Alan was somehow able to resist his hypnotic suggestions, as clearly the *Snoozeslumber* was too big to be underneath his swim cap. So Sammy did something he had never done before. He used black ops hypnosis. It is a very secret, but very real way to put someone into such a *deep, hypnotic, sleep* that only three people in the world knew how to do.

Sammy whispered the magical hypnotic words he needed to say in order to control Alan's mind: *'As you sleep zenfully in the Zenflo you begin to allow my voice and the spaces between my words to take you deeper and deeper into sleep. Sleepier now in this very moment, more sleepy than you have ever been in your entire life* **(P)**. As you float there in that tank you'll notice now there is a door in your mind labelled "Top Secret Zone". Open the door and enter into the top secret zone. Notice all of your secrets are stored here. Look around and see where the secret of the *Snoozeslumber* 2000 is kept. Your mission is to tell me on the count of three where you are seeing that *Snoozeslumber* 2000. One. Two. Three.'

Alan immediately blurted out, 'It's hidden in the boot of my *sleepmobile*.' Sammy immediately locked Alan into the *Zenflo* and turned the temperature to freezing cold. As he ran out of the *Zenflo Hypnolagoon* he could hear Alan shrieking at the shock of being woken by the chilly water. Sammy found Alan's *sleepmobile* in the car park at the back of the *hypnolagoon*.

Alan's *sleepmobile* is a crazy invention – it is a self-driving car which allows *you to sleep, easily and comfortably,* while getting you to your destination. Its sleek and aerodynamic style ensures you don't feel any lumps or bumps on your journey. The dimly lit purple interior is designed to create a *super-cosy atmosphere which will help you drift away into a deep, deep sleep* **(P)**. The *super soft* seats recline into *beds* which are at the exact temperature to help *you drift away*. As the car is driving, beautiful music plays and *you hear soft sounds* like the crashing of waves on the seashore or the gentle whispers of wind to help *you drift and float away, floating and drifting, drifting and floating.*

You can control everything – the temperature, the volume of the music, and the speed of the car itself – with only your mind. Imagine now what it would be like to be inside the *sleepmobile* and *allow yourself to relax into the wonderful magic of the sleepiest car you've ever been in, inside your mind* **(P)**.

Sammy picked the lock on the *sleepmobile* and jumped inside. He knew he had only seconds to programme the satellite navigation to bring him to the theatre before he *fell sound asleep. The moment he plugged in the address he began to yawn. Yawn after yawn, he must have yawned a thousand times. With every yawn his eyes felt heavier and heavier. His body relaxed deeper and deeper* **(P)**. The sound of the sea from the speakers washed over his entire body like a soothing lullaby, drowning out any sound from the external world. Sammy enjoyed the restful, rejuvenating slumber until he arrived at the front of the theatre.

He opened the boot and sure enough there was the *Snoozeslumber 2000*. He grabbed it and ran into the theatre where all one hundred people were still *sleeping soundly*. They all *looked so calm and peaceful*. Although Alan had put them to sleep without their permission they were *enjoying the deep rest* they were getting. Sammy knew if he woke them abruptly they might get a fright, so he programmed the *Snoozeslumber 2000* to wake them really gently. He aimed it at them and hit the button. They all slowly opened their eyes and gently returned back to normal, with smiles beaming across their faces. Although Alan had put them to sleep without their permission they all had actually *enjoyed being asleep*. Sammy hugged each and every one of them as they exited the theatre. As for Alan, he was still stuck with his rubber chicken, freezing in the *Zenflo Hypnolagoon*.

The sleepy people realised how good it had been for them to get such *deep, powerful sleep, just as you are about to now.*

As you snuggle into your cosy bed, imagine you have your own personal Snoozeslumber 2000. Imagine what it looks and feels like **(P)**. Imagine it has the magical power to help whisk you away into the world of your dreams. *Allow the soft glow and the gentle hum guide you into a calm, deep sleep. With every breath you take from this moment on you fill your entire body with relaxation. With every breath you let go you find any tightness in your body just disappears. Inhaling deep relaxation. Exhaling tension* **(P)**.

You are now an artist and your mind is your canvas. Use your *Snoozeslumber 2000* to begin to *paint positive thoughts, pictures, dreams, ideas and concepts inside the walls of your mind.* Enjoy these thoughts as you allow yourself to *drift away into a deep, deep sleep. Sleepier and sleepier, deeper and deeper* **(P)**.

You'll notice now my voice getting *lower and lower as you slip into a deep sleep easily and quickly.* Become very absorbed now in your mind as your entire body slows down in preparation for sleep. Allow yourself to drift from dream to dream easily and peacefully, enjoying this wonderful night's sleep. *Now with every breath you take you find you feel twice as relaxed* **(P)**.

And now in your mind imagine you are inside your own private sleepmobile. Sit inside and notice the seats are *so cosy* they are like sitting on a giant marshmallow. Allow the seat to recline back so *you* are in a *sleep* position inside the car. As the car moves you enter into a sleep tunnel. This magical tunnel is filled with all kinds of things to help *you drift into sleep.* As you travel through this endless tunnel you feel my love for you and you feel more safe than you have ever felt before. You notice now there are numbers in the ceiling, coloured purple. These numbers start at 1,000. *With every number you count down from 1,000 you find you relax even more. Sleepier and sleepier with every number you see, deeper and deeper you go* **(P)**. One thousand down to 999, *the better you feel the more you will allow yourself to sleep and the more you allow yourself to sleep the better you feel* **(P)**. Nine hundred and ninety-eight, relaxing even more. Continue to count the numbers now as you relax and drift away right here, right now …

ACKNOWLEDGEMENTS

I would like to thank Claire for her dedication and assistance in helping put my crazy thoughts on paper in a hopefully understandable manner.

Thanks to Sarah, Aoibheann and the team in Gill books for not running for the hills when I suggested this book to them. Your support and guidance are much appreciated.

Thanks to my mum and dad – Ken and Kitty – for being the soundest parents anyone could have. You're absolute legends.

Thanks to Braden, Breanna and Mairead for putting up with having an oddball for a dad and husband and not running away!

NOTES

1 Raymann, R. J., Swaab, D. F., & Van Someren, E. J. (2007). Skin temperature and sleep-onset latency: Changes with age and insomnia. *Physiology & Behavior*, 90(2–3), 257–266, https://doi.org/10.1016/j.physbeh.2006.09.008

2 Scullin, M. K., Krueger, M. L., Ballard, H. K., Pruett, N., & Bliwise, D. L. (2018). The effects of bedtime writing on difficulty falling asleep: A polysomnographic study comparing to-do lists and completed activity lists. *Journal of Experimental Psychology: General*, 147(1), 139–146, <https://doi.org/10.1037/xge0000374>.

3 Chennaoui, M., Vanneau, T., Trignol, A., Arnal, P. J., Gomez-Merino, D., Baudot, C., Perez, J. M., Pochettino, S., Eirale, C., & Chalabi, H. (2021). How does sleep help recovery from exercise-induced muscle injuries? *Journal of Science and*

Medicine in Sport, 24(10), 982–987, <https://doi.org/10.1016/j.jsams.2021.05.007>.

4   Chang, A. M., Aeschbach, D., Duffy, J. F., & Czeisler, C. A. (2014). Evening use of light-emitting eReaders negatively affects sleep, circadian timing, and next-morning alertness. *Proceedings of the National Academy of Sciences of the United States of America*, 112(4), 1232–1237, <https://doi.org/10.1073/pnas.1418490112>.

5   Harding, E. C., Franks, N. P., & Wisden, W. (2019). The temperature dependence of sleep. *Frontiers in Neuroscience*, 13, <https://doi.org/10.3389/fnins.2019.00336>.

6   Harmat, L., Takács, J., & Bódizs, R. (2008). Music improves sleep quality in students. *Journal of Advanced Nursing*, 62(3), 327–335, <https://doi.org/10.1111/j.1365-2648.2008.04602.x>.

7   Manoogian, E. N., & Panda, S. (2017). Circadian rhythms, time-restricted feeding, and healthy aging. *Ageing Research Reviews*, 39, 59–67, https://doi.org/10.1016/j.arr.2016.12.006

8   Pigeon, W. R., Carr, M., Gorman, C., & Perlis, M. L. (2010). Effects of a tart cherry juice beverage on the sleep of older adults with insomnia: A pilot study. *Journal of Medicinal Food*, 13(3), 579–583, <https://doi.org/10.1089/jmf.2009.0096>.

9   Howatson, G., Bell, P. G., Tallent, J., Middleton, B., McHugh, M. P., & Ellis, J. (2011). Effect of tart cherry juice (*Prunus cerasus*) on melatonin levels and enhanced sleep quality. *European Journal of Nutrition*, 51(8), 909–916, <https://doi.org/10.1007/s00394-011-0263-7>.

10 Verde, A., Míguez, J. M., Leão, J. M., Gago-Martínez, A., & Gallardo, M. (2022). Melatonin content in walnuts and other commercial nuts. Influence of cultivar, ripening

and processing (roasting). *Journal of Food Composition and Analysis*, 105, 104180, <https://doi.org/10.1016/j.jfca.2021.104180>.

11   Lin, H. H., Tsai, P. S., Fang, S. C., & Liu, J. F. (2011). Effect of kiwifruit consumption on sleep quality in adults with sleep problems. *Asia Pacific Journal of Clinical Nutrition*, 20(2), 169–174, <https://pubmed.ncbi.nlm.nih.gov/21669584>.

12   Doherty, R., Madigan, S. M., Nevill, A. M., Warrington, G. D., & Ellis, J. (2023). The impact of kiwifruit consumption on the sleep and recovery of elite athletes. *Nutrients*, 15(10), 2274, <https://doi.org/10.3390/nu15102274>.

13   Bermingham, K., Stensrud, S., Asnicar, F., Valdes, A., Franks, P. W., Wolf, J., Hadjigeorgiou, G., Davies, R., Spector, T. D., Segata, N., Berry, S., & Hall, W. (2023). Exploring the relationship between social jetlag with gut microbial composition, diet and cardiometabolic health, in the ZOE PREDICT 1 cohort. *European Journal of Nutrition*, 62(8), 3135–3147, <https://doi.org/10.1007/s00394-023-03204-x>.

14   Roy, C., Kurilshikov, A., Leeming, E. R., Visconti, A., Bowyer, R. C. E., Menni, C., Falchi, M., Koutníková, H., Veiga, P., Zhernakova, A., Derrien, M., & Spector, T. D. (2022). Yoghurt consumption is associated with changes in the composition of the human gut microbiome and metabolome. *BMC Microbiology*, 22(1), <https://doi.org/10.1186/s12866-021-02364-2>.

15   Fukushige, H., Fukuda, Y., Tanaka, M., Inami, K., Wada, K., Tsumura, Y., Kondo, M., Harada, T., Wakamura, T., & Morita, T. (2014). Effects of tryptophan-rich breakfast and light exposure during the daytime on melatonin secretion at

night. *Journal of Physiological Anthropology*, 33(1), <https://doi.org/10.1186/1880-6805-33-33>.

16 Montgomery, P., Burton, J. R., Sewell, R. P., Spreckelsen, T. F., & Richardson, A. J. (2014). Fatty acids and sleep in UK children: Subjective and pilot objective sleep results from the DOLAB study – a randomized controlled trial. *Journal of Sleep Research*, 8 March, <https://doi.org/10.1111/jsr.12135>.

17 Simon, E. B., Rossi, A., Harvey, A. G., & Walker, M. P. (2019). Overanxious and underslept. *Nature Human Behaviour*, 4(1), 100–110, <https://doi.org/10.1038/s41562-019-0754-8>.

18 Leproult, R., Copinschi, G., Buxton, O., & Van Cauter, E. (1997). Sleep loss results in an elevation of cortisol levels the next evening. *Sleep*, 20(10), 865–870, <https://pubmed.ncbi.nlm.nih.gov/9415946/#:~:text=After%20partial%20and%20total%20sleep,by%20at%20least%201%20hour>.

19 Clark, B. C., Mahato, N. K., Nakazawa, M., Law, T., & Thomas, J. S. (2014). The power of the mind: The cortex as a critical determinant of muscle strength/weakness. *Journal of Neurophysiology*, 112(12), 3219–3226, <https://doi.org/10.1152/jn.00386.2014>.

20 Cohen, S., Janicki-Deverts, D., Turner, R. B., & Doyle, W. J. (2014). Does hugging provide stress-buffering social support? A study of susceptibility to upper respiratory infection and illness. *Psychological Science*, 26(2), 135–147, <https://doi.org/10.1177/0956797614559284>.

21 Chamine, I., Atchley, R., & Oken, B. (2018). Hypnosis intervention effects on sleep outcomes: A systematic review. *Journal of Clinical Sleep Medicine*, 14(02), 271–283, <https://doi.org/10.5664/jcsm.6952>.

22 *Science Daily* (2014, 14 June). Hypnosis extends restorative slow-wave sleep, research shows, <https://www.sciencedaily.com/releases/2014/06/140602101207.htm>.

23 Naselaris, T., Olman, C. A., Stansbury, D., Uğurbil, K., & Gallant, J. L. (2015). A voxel-wise encoding model for early visual areas decodes mental images of remembered scenes. *NeuroImage, 105*, 215–228, <https://doi.org/10.1016/j.neuroimage.2014.10.018>.

24 Nguyen, J., & Brymer, E. (2018). Nature-based guided imagery as an intervention for state anxiety. *Frontiers in Psychology, 9*, <https://doi.org/10.3389/fpsyg.2018.01858>.

25 Martin, E., Ressler, K. J., Binder, E. B., & Nemeroff, C. B. (2009). The neurobiology of anxiety disorders: Brain imaging, genetics, and psychoneuroendocrinology. *Psychiatric Clinics of North America, 32*(3), 549–575, <https://doi.org/10.1016/j.psc.2009.05.004>.

26 Lee, S., Charles, S. T., & Almeida, D. M. (2020). Change is good for the brain: Activity diversity and cognitive functioning across adulthood. *Journals of Gerontology*: Series B, 76(6), 1036–1048, <https://doi.org/10.1093/geronb/gbaa020>.

27 Epton, T., & Harris, P. R. (2008). Self-affirmation promotes health behavior change. *Health Psychology, 27*(6), 746–752, <https://doi.org/10.1037/0278-6133.27.6.746>.

28 Shimoda, S., Shimoda, M., & Higuchi, O. (2022). Effect of self-affirmation on smartphone use reduction among heavy users. *Psychological Reports, 126*(3), 1362–1377, <https://doi.org/10.1177/00332941211069514>.

29 Dutcher, J. M., Creswell, J. D., Pacilio, L. E., Harris, P. R., Klein, W. M. P., Levine, J. M., Bower, J. E., Muscatell, K. A., &

Eisenberger, N. I. (2016). Self-affirmation activates the ventral striatum. *Psychological Science, 27*(4), 455–466, <https://doi.org/10.1177/0956797615625989>.

30 Lee, Y., Lu, C., Cheng, W., & Li, H. (2022). The impact of mouth-taping in mouth-breathers with mild obstructive sleep apnea: A preliminary study. *Healthcare, 10*(9), 1755, <https://doi.org/10.3390/healthcare10091755>.

31 Greengross, G., Silvia, P. J., & Crasson, S. J. (2023). Psychotic and autistic traits among magicians and their relationship with creative beliefs. *British Journal of Psychiatry Open, 9*(6), <https://doi.org/10.1192/bjo.2023.609>.

32 De Vries, S., Verheij, R., & Groenewegen, P. (2003). Natural environments – healthy environments? An exploratory analysis of the relationship between greenspace and health. *Environment and Planning A: Economy and Space, 35*(10), 1717–1731, <https://doi.org/10.1068/a35111>.

33 Buck, D. (2016). *Gardens and Health: Implications for Policy and Practice.* The King's Fund, <https://www.kingsfund.org.uk/insight-and-analysis/reports/gardens-health>.

34 Chalmin-Pui, L.S., Griffiths, A., Roe, J., Heaton, T., & Cameron, R. (2021). Why garden? Attitudes and the perceived benefits of home gardening. *Cities, 112,* <https://www.sciencedirect.com/science/article/pii/S0264275121000160>.

35 Li, Q., Ochiai, H., Ochiai, T., Takayama, N., Kumeda, S., Miura, T., Aoyagi, Y., & Imai, M. (2022). Effects of forest bathing (shinrin-yoku) on serotonin in serum, depressive symptoms and subjective sleep quality in middle-aged males. *Environmental Health and Preventive Medicine, 27*(0), 44, <https://doi.org/10.1265/ehpm.22-00136>.

36 Sokal, K., & Sokal, P. (2011). Earthing the human body influences physiologic processes. *Journal of Alternative and Complementary Medicine, 17*(4), 301–308, <https://doi.org/10.1089/acm.2010.0687>.

37 Ghaly, M., & Teplitz, D. (2004). The biologic effects of grounding the human body during sleep as measured by cortisol levels and subjective reporting of sleep, pain, and stress. *Journal of Alternative and Complementary Medicine, 10*(5), 767–776, <https://doi.org/10.1089/acm.2004.10.767>.

38 Feinstein, J. S., Khalsa, S. S., Yeh, H. W., Wohlrab, C., Simmons, W. K., Stein, M. B., & Paulus, M. P. (2018). Examining the short-term anxiolytic and antidepressant effect of Floatation-REST. *PloS one, 13*(2), e0190292, <https://doi.org/10.1371/journal.pone.0190292>.

39 Oesterling, C. F., Borg, C., Juhola, E., & Lancel, M. (2023). The influence of sexual activity on sleep: A diary study. *Journal of Sleep Research, 32*(4), <https://doi.org/10.1111/jsr.13814>.